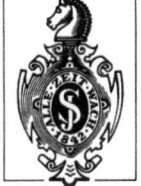

H. Schams · J. Bretscher

Ultrasonographic Diagnosis in Obstetrics and Gynecology

Ultraschalldiagnose in Geburtshilfe und Gynäkologie

Echographie en obstétrique et gynécologie

Diagnostico con ultrasonido en obstetricia y ginecologia

La diagnosi ecografica a ultrasuoni nell'ostetricia e nella ginecologia

Springer-Verlag
Berlin Heidelberg New York 1975

Dr. med. HOSSEIN SCHAMS
Prof. Dr. med. JÜRG BRETSCHER

Maternité Inselhof Triemli,
Klinik für Geburtsmedizin und Gynäkologie, CH-8063 Zurich

With 140 Figures

ISBN-13: 978-3-642-66135-8   e-ISBN-13: 978-3-642-66133-4
DOI: 10.1007/978-3-642-66133-4

Library of Congress Cataloging in Publication Data. SCHAMS, HOSSEIN, 1942–
Ultrasonographic diagnosis in obstetrics and gynecology. Bibliography: p.
Includes index. 1. Diagnosis, Ultrasonic. 2. Obstetrics. 3. Gynecology. I. BRETSCHER,
JÜRG., joint author. II. Title. III. Title: Ultraschalldiagnose in Geburtshilfe und
Gynäkologie. [DNLM: 1. Gynecologic diseases—diagnosis. 2. Pregnancy compli-
cations—Diagnosis. 3. Prenatal diagnosis. 4. Ultrasonics—diagnostic use. WQ202
S299u] RG107.5.U4S3   618   75-8787

© by Springer-Verlag Berlin Heidelberg 1975.
Softcover reprint of the hardcover 1st edition 1975

Typesetting, printing, and bookbinding by Universitätsdruckerei H. Stürtz AG,
Würzburg

Preface

To day ultrasonic diagnosis holds a firm place in the field of perinatal medicine. Its absence from the equipment of a modern obstetric clinic, where recognition and evaluation of pregnancies at risk is a particular concern, is inconceivable. In routine operation ultrasonics mainly comprises the diagnosis of retardation of fetal growth—primarily in the case of placental insufficiency, and also in location of the placenta.

Since the pioneer work, which in the German-speaking countries was carried out chiefly by Kratochwil, various working groups have established themselves at numerous hospitals and are endeavouring to strengthen the clinical credibility of ultrasonic diagnosis. The great advances in the future, however, will be made in the field of technical equipment: we hope that engineers will soon provide us with refinements in handling and with new contrast processes (grey scale and color diagnosis), to be used in routine operation.

The examples shown have been selected from our two years of experience. Whenever possible, the results have been compared and checked with clinical and laboratory methods. For instance, the biparietal diameter, measured before delivery, was remeasured with calipers when infants were born by Caesarian section; most cases of placenta praevia and posterior-wall placenta have been confirmed by manual detachment of the placenta or by Caesarian section; all vesicular moles have been examined histologically.

We have been working since 1971 with equipment manufactured by the Picker Corporation, Cleveland, Ohio 44143, USA.

Overrating a single method will never lead to the expected clinical successes. The relationship of ultrasonic diagnosis to all other methods of perinatal diagnosis is that of mutual adjuvants. Especially in the field of obstetric prophylaxis and diagnosis, history and clinical examination take precedence over any one possible apparatus or biochemical method.

Zurich, March 1975 J. BRETSCHER
H. SCHAMS

Contents

Abbreviations, see fold-out table inside back cover

Introduction

Ultrasound consists of waves of frequency above 18,000 Hz and hence outside the audible range. Sound is audible in the frequency range 16 to 18,000 Hz; below 16 Hz one speaks of infrasound or subsonic vibrations.

Ultrasonics came into prominence for locating submarines; it is used in oceanographic research for sounding ocean depths, and in industry for testing materials. Ultrasonic diagnosis was introduced in obstetrics and gynecology in 1958 by EDLER and HERTZ. It is a relatively simple method of examination that can be applied at any time without preparation and without adverse effects on the patient. Investigations carried out so far have shown that, provided the test conditions really correspond to the power levels used in diagnosis, ultrasonics is without danger for mother and child.

The crystal formations of piezo-electric crystals (e.g. quartz and barium titanate) become elastic under the influence of an electric field, i.e. they are deformed reversibly and thus generate ultrasonic waves. This effect was observed in 1880 by the CURIES. Conversely, ultrasonic waves, on striking the crystal, cause electrical polarization phenomena, that can be displayed on an oscillograph. Because of this property, a piezo-electric crystal can thus serve as both transmitter and receiver: first it is supplied with electrical pulses from a control unit. Then during a short subsequent restperiod it becomes capable of recording a reflected pressure wave. The piezo-electric crystal, which is located in the probe head of the ultrasonic instrument, alternates its transmitting and receiving function at microsecond intervals. From this alternating function the term *Pulse-Echo Method* is derived. The echo can be displayed in one or more dimensions by means of an oscillograph and can be photographed. Single-dimensional recordings are known as an A-scan, multidimensional records a a B-scan.

The echo is produced on the basis of the following principles. High-frequency sound waves approximately follow the laws for electromagnetic waves. For ultrasonic diagnosis, the law, well-known from optics, is of particular importance; this states that, when a sound beam passes from one medium into another medium of different optical density, part of the energy is reflected. A new echo occurs each time the part of the energy, that is not reflected and is propagated further in the tissue in the original direction of the sound passes into another medium.

The pulse-echo method must be distinguished from the *continuous-wave method* using the *Doppler effect,* incorrectly known, for short, as the Doppler method. The term "continuous-wave" has nothing to do with the length of time taken for the examination, but signifies that there is no alternation of the two functions of *one* crystal, as explained above. One crystal continuously transmits sound waves and a second crystal serves as the receiver. The frequencies of the sound waves are changed at *medium boundaries* (boundary surfaces) which move parallel to the direction of the sound. The reflected waves that excite the receiver crystal have a different frequency. This interference can be made audible. The continuous-wave method is eminently suitable for short or long-term monitoring of fetal heart beats. The moving medium, which is responsible for the Doppler effect, is formed by the myocardium.

Our illustrated guide is chiefly concerned with the pulse-echo method.

A-Scan · Amplitude Diagram · Notch Diagram · One-Dimensional Diagram

The main application of the A-scan technique in obstetrics is for the measurement of the biparietal diameter of the fetal head. From this parameter conclusions can be drawn concerning the size and weight of the fetus (Fig. I, p. 2).

Conclusions concerning the gestation period are permissible, provided there are no indications of retardation of growth (placental insufficiency). The amplitude diagram is accurate to ± 2 mm. It is essential to identify the so-called central echo. When the test probe is applied above the pubic symphysis, peaks or groups of peaks are visible (Fig. II, p. 3).

Besides the central echo, further peaks can occur between peaks B_1 and B_2; these are known as lateral reflections and originate from the lateral ventricles or temporal horns. The central echo can be caused by the falx cerebri, the septum pellucidum, the third ventricle or the epiphysis. The disadvantage of the procedure is that it is relatively time-consuming, because it is necessary to find the greatest distance between the front and rear parietal bones. Comparison with a B-scan taken at the same time or immediately afterwards improves interpretation and accuracy.

A special form of the A-scan is the *Time motion* or M-method, where the reflections arise from moving boundary surfaces.

B-Scan · Light-Spot Image · Two-Dimensional Image

Instead of a stationary test probe, a moving crystal is used to visualize the organ in question. The reflected sound waves are displayed not as spikes but as light-spots and are recorded photographically, thus producing, as it were, anatomical cross-

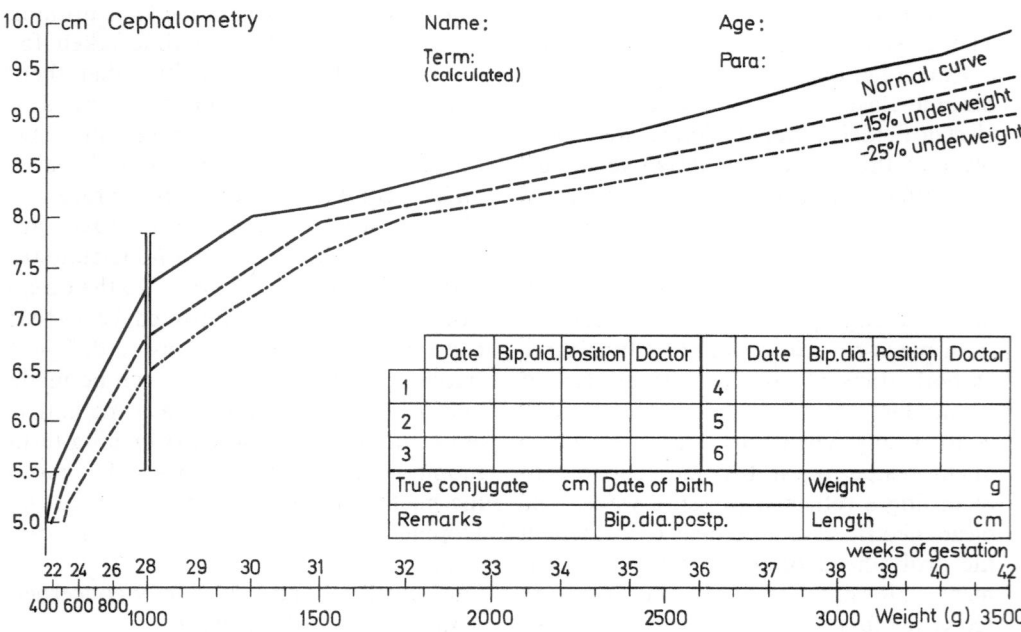

Fig. I. Nomogram for determining the fetal body weight and the gestation age from the biparietal diameter. Modified according to HANSMANN, M.: Arch. Gynäk. **211**, 264 (1971)

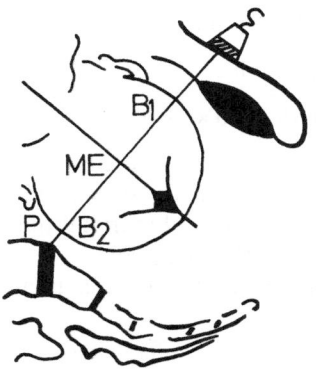
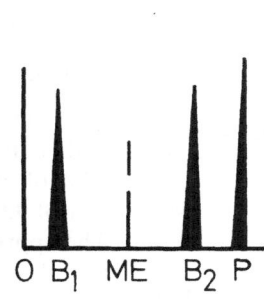

sections. Besides the fetal cranium, it becomes possible to visualize the placenta, uterus, fetal cavities, thorax, small members and, in gynecological diagnosis, also tumors, the liver, kidneys, and other organs.

When ultrasonic waves pass from a gaseous to a liquid medium, practically all the waves are reflected. For this reason, liquid coupling by Vaseline, oil, or a gel-like fluid is necessary in all the methods mentioned. We use Aquasonic 100.

Evidence of Early Pregnancy

(see Fig. 1, p. 14)

When the pregnant uterus is still small and its fundus has not yet risen above the level of the symphysis, the bony structure of the symphysis and the external sex organs form an obstacle to the location of the uterus. For this reason, the examination is always carried out with a full, almost overfull, bladder and with the pelvis slightly raised. This forces the uterus upward, and the air-filled intestinal loops, which have poor sound conduction, move outside the sound field. Thus the embryo can be visualized with a B-scan from 7 weeks of gestation, although it does not determine whether the fetus is alive, a

question that has to be decided by repeated HCG determinations.

Of course the life of the infant can also be detected in early pregnancy with the aid of ultrasonic diagnosis, by detecting either heart action or fetal movement. With the abdominal sound head, heart actions can be detected from the 13th week of gestation. In principle, recording can be carried out with the A- or M-scan (The continuous-wave method also makes abdominal reception of heart action possible from the 13th week). With special techniques, which are not dealt with in our guide, heart actions can be detected as early as the 8th to 10th week. These involve the use of vaginal sound heads or of rotating directional transmitters with a reflector optical system, included in models by other manufacturers. The detection of heart action at such an early point in time is probably a matter of the reception of movements that are communicated to the surrounding organs (umbilical cord, uterine wall) from the heart. With directional transmitters, fetal movements can also be detected from the 8th week of pregnancy.

The fetal cranium, which is indeed of particular importance, can be shown with the B-scan from the 13th week of pregnancy. Indeed, the biparietal diameter can be approximately located only when an elliptical shape of the head can be shown, but this distance only becomes certain when the central echo is detected.

Determining the Biparietal Diameter

(see Figs. 2–11, p. 17)

A graph on page 7 points out the relationship between biparietal diameter and weight.

Most significant is the detecting of retardation in the growth of the child (small-for-date baby, development deficiency). Further, this method is advantageous when duration of the pregnancy is uncertain, in such cases such as rhesus incompatibility, diabetes, or EPH syndrome, in which the viability of the fetus has to be considered.

The biparietal diameter permits us to estimate the weight with a reliability of ±400 g, when working with a measurement accuracy of ±2 mm. The weight prognosis becomes more accurate, namely ±200 g, if the thorax diameter is taken into account; but this obviously causes more technical difficulties. Even more exact prognoses are probably possible by correlating the biparietal diameter to the thorax diameter.

In principle, either method A or B can be used, but we prefer the B-scan. The fetal skull is located and the whole circumference of the head, with the indispensible central echo, is plotted by moving around it with the sound head. The greatest transverse distance of the cranium corresponds to the biparietal diameter. Then, as a matter of routine, we plot an A-scan that serves as a check on the B-scan. Here, too, the central echo (central peak) is indispensible.

Besides using graphical nomograms, we can calculate the weight of the child either by THOMPSON's formula:

Weight = 1 060 × Bip. dia. — 6 575

or a simpler formula:

Weight = Bip. dia. — 6 × 1 000

The weight of the child exceeds 2 500 g with a biparietal diameter of 8.5 cm in 80% of cases and with a biparietal diameter of 9.0 cm in 91% of cases.

The approximate length can be estimated as follows:

Length (cm) = Bip. dia. × $5^1/_2$

On the average, the biparietal diameter measures 9.3 cm at full term.

Monitoring Fetal Growth

(see Figs. 12–26, p. 30)

Ultrasonics is very useful in elucidating discrepancies between amenorrhoea and the weight of the child. In such discrepancies, a single measurement of the biparietal diameter is of some importance; but monitoring of the growth at weekly intervals is more meaningful. In undisturbed pregnancies, the increase in biparietal diameter from the 20th to the 40th week of pregnancy is 1.6 mm per week. Repeated weekly examinations are undertaken if clinical anamnestic pointers indicate possible placental insufficiency (EPH syndrome) or if the conventional external examination suggests a "small baby". It is advisable to determine endocrine parameters in the 24-hour urine or serum, combined with cardiotocography and in later pregnancy with amnioscopy.

Hydrocephalus can also be diagnosed.

For monitoring growth, we use the B-scan in the first half of pregnancy and both the A-scan and B-scan in the second half. If, in exceptional cases, we wish to detect a growth trend in early pregnancy, when the head can still not be located, we measure the uterine cavity.

Detection of the Fetal Heart Action

(see Figs. 27–31, p. 38)

Ultrasonic diagnosis was introduced in cardiology by EDLER and HERTZ in 1954. It is possible, in adults, to diagnose tricuspid and mitral-valve defects and determine the thickness of the myocardium and pericardial exudation.

As mentioned on page 1, the Doppler (continuous-wave) method is preferred for the routing monitoring of the fetal heart frequency. Heart action can, however, also be represented in principle with an A- or M-scan. For the earliest time of detection, see page 3.

With the aid of the time–motion method (M-scan), heart movements can be displayed as curves and photographed; it is not known which of the two ventricular valves we detect. Often the contractions are also visible on the wall of the heart or the large vessels; they also can be recorded as transmitted pulsations of adjacent organs.

Analyses of the shape of the curves and possible conclusions on hypoxia or vitiation of the heart are still in a very early stage.

Anterior-Wall Placenta

(see Figs. 32–47, p. 44)

Ultrasonic placentography serves well in locating the placenta. It is used before transabdominal amniocentesis to monitor rhesus incompatibility (determination of the bilirubinoids in the amniotic fluid) or to estimate maturity of the lungs by determination of the lecithin and sphyngomyeline in the amniotic fluid. Locating the placenta is equally important in dealing with possible hemorrhages in the second half of pregnancy (placenta praevia, malposition).

Placental location by ultrasonics, if performed by experienced hands, is equal in value to isotope tracing. Isotope tracing is carried out by injecting into the mother radioactively labeled serum proteins with a short half-life.

These two methods have replaced X-ray and thermal location, which were sometimes not without danger and, above all, less reliable.

In principle, the location of the placenta can also be approximated with the continuous-wave (Doppler) method. However, this method gives unsatisfactory results because a differential diagnosis between anterior-wall and posterior-wall placenta cannot be carried out; also, no decision can be made on the extent of the placenta because the boundary cannot be detected. The A-scan method has also been tried with little success. The B-scan method is the preferred one. With this method it is possible to detect the full extent of the placenta and its boundary.

Posterior-Wall Placenta

(see Figs. 48–55, p. 64)

According to data by HOFBAUER, the frequency of occurrence of the posterior-wall and posterior–lateral-wall placenta is 34%. Locating it is not difficult with our equipment, even in obese patients, since by setting the appropriate amplification and depth compensation, a penetration depth of the sound waves up to 30 cm can be achieved.

One special feature that deserves attention in the location of the posterior-wall placenta is the occurrence of echo-free regions. These appear on the oscillograph or in photographs as empty spaces and can restrict decision as to the extent of the placenta, if they happen to be in the edge region of the placenta. These extinction phenomena occur because parts of the child (head, torso, extremities) reabsorb the weak echos reflected from the placenta behind them. In certain cases, a posterior-wall placenta can only be determined by the echo-free region.

Fundal Placenta

(see Figs. 56–59, p. 74)

Locating the placenta that lies mainly in the fundus also causes no difficulty. A longitudinal section in the median plane shows its full extent, and a transition to a posterior-wall placenta can be made visible by amplification and depth compensation.

Regarding placenta location in general, we must mention that recognition is not possible before the 16th week of pregnancy. Besides location, thickness naturally also has to be assessed. If weekly checks show a rapid increase in thickness, this is an indication of hydrops of the fetus and placenta. Thus, ultrasonic diagnosis also forms a useful adjunct in supervising rhesus incompatibility, in which spectrophotometry of the amniotic fluid, of course takes first place.

Placenta Praevia

(see Figs. 60–70, p. 80)

The prerequisite for diagnosis of placenta praevia is the location of the internal orifice of the uterus. 30 to 60 minutes before examination to plot a sectional diagram, the patient should drink half a liter of tea. In this way a tightly filled bladder is achieved and the lower section of the uterus becomes visible.

According to their definitions, the diagnoses of placenta praevia partialis (lateralis), marginalis, and totalis refer to an orifice of the uterus which is opened 3 to 5 cm. This classification is based on findings by palpation. Ultrasonic diagnosis for placental location is indeed carried out for the most part during pregnancy, that is with the orifice closed. The result of this is that differentiation between placenta praevia partialis and placenta praevia marginalis cannot be clearly carried out. On the other hand, placenta praevia totalis can be diagnosed with certainty because the placenta can be seen in its full extent.

It is often surprising that the placenta praevia extends a long way toward the fundus. In many cases the placenta is conspicuously thin. In the literature, mistaken diagnoses are said to amount to 3 to 6%.

Premature Detachment of the Normally Located Placenta

(see Figs. 71 and 72, p. 96)

For routine clinical purposes, ultrasonic diagnosis plays a very subsidiary role in this clinical picture. The clinical picture itself stands in the foreground of the diagnosis: History of bleeding, sometimes more or less sudden sensation of pain, tension of the uterus (basic tone), irritability of the uterus; perhaps a disturbance of coagulation in the sense of hypo- or afibrinogenemia. Nevertheless, we would like to present below an interesting case of a total premature detachment.

This is the case of a 22-year-old primipara, in whom labor was induced 24 hours after premature rupture of the membranes. The first discrete sign was a change of the heart frequency to the silent oscillation type without decelerations, and after changing to the lateral position a restricted undulatory oscillation type. 50 minutes after commencement of induction, there was a sudden drop in heart rate with severe pain; the uterus distended. The fetus died quickly. Spontaneous birth did not occur until $8^1/_2$ hours after the acute attack.

The pictures show a totally detached anterior-wall placenta, and between placenta and the anterior wall of the uterus an echo-free zone 3 cm wide, which was caused by accumulation of retroplacental blood.

Twins

(see Figs. 73–79, p. 100)

For years we have carried out the B-scan plot when there is clinical suspicion of twins, primarily to verify the diagnosis. Ultrasonic diagnosis, which permits certain diagnosis with little time expenditure, should be used on a liberal scale because twin pregnancies and births count as a risk: $^2/_3$ of all twin pregnancies end before the 39th week; the proportion of premature births is increased, while the average weight of the children is only 2,700 g. Perinatal mortality and morbidity is increased. If we also consider the fact that in multiple pregnancies the incidence of an EPH syndrome is multiplied and thus a double risk arises, the importance of detecting twin pregnancies as early as possible before full term becomes clear. Through the primary use of ultrasonic diagnosis, radiography can be reduced to a minimum. X-ray examination is suggested if: clinical suspicion still exists, ultrasonic diagnosis is made difficult in very obese mothers, or pronounced edema of the abdominal wall or massive hydramnios occur. The proof of twins is based on the representation of two crania. If the heads are located, the position of the fetuses can be determined.

Vesicular Moles

(see Figs. 80–86, p. 108)

Ultrasonics is an extraordinarily reliable method for the diagnosis of the vesicular mole. We have already relied on it in a rare case with repeated normal chorion gonadotropin values. The ultrasonic image (B-scan) is characterized by a snow flake-like "filling" of the cavum uteri ("snowstorm"). The echos, in the form of dots and dashes, mostly arise from the cyst walls of the individual vesicles.

We use ultrasonic diagnosis to determine whether a vesicular mole exists in the case of:
— Discrepancy between amenorrhoea and uterus size in early pregnancy.
— Conspicuously relaxed uterus.
— Persistent or intermittent bleeding from the 4th to the 20th week of pregnancy without sign of an ordinary abortion.
— Absence of evidence of heart action (Doppler method) from the 13th week.

Naturally, the examination will be combined with the semi-quantitative determination of the chorion-gonadotropins. In this connection, however, ultrasonic diagnosis assumes particular importance when the rate is high, because a differential diagnosis must be made to determine if it is a twin pregnancy or whether these are the higher limiting values of a normal single pregnancy.

Hydramnios

(see Figs. 87–89, p. 118)

The term hydramnios is used if the quantity of amniotic fluid is more than 2 liters. If, due to an above-average abdominal circumference, a differential diagnosis must be made to distinguish this from a twin pregnancy, ultrasonic diagnosis provides clarification in two respects (see "Twins", page 7). In rare cases the situation also arises, in other than an intra-uterine pregnancy, that the suspected hydramnios are recognised as an ovarian cyst or ascites. In addition to ideopathic hydramnios, usually characterized by rapid progress and caused by an unknown change in the function of the chorion epithelium, an excessive quantity of amniotic fluid is found in abnormalities and diseases of the fetus (twins, anencephalus and spina bifida, oesophagus atresia) and in diseases of the mother (diabetes, syphilis).

The ultrasonic image is characterized by a broad intra-uterine region which is echo-free and uniform, corresponding to the amniotic fluid.

Intra-Uterine Death of the Fetus

(see Figs. 90–95, p. 122)

Ultrasonic diagnosis makes it possible to approach the death of the embryo from all diagnostic aspects except the endocrine parameters. The Doppler method as well as the time–motion method (M-scan) permit the absence of heart action to be recorded. Of course, the examination must be carried out several times on different days. With the B-scan technique it is possible to detect typical signs, such as those obtained from X-ray diagnosis: the "roof-tile"-like displacement of the cranial bones (Spalding's sign); the (often pouch-like) deformation of the cranium (collection-bag sign); the occurrence of an intermediate gap between the scalp and the cranium (Halo, nimbus). The so-called radiographic vertebral signs (gibbus and abnormal lateral curvature) are considerably less easy to show by ultrasonic diagnosis.

Using ultrasonic equipment with rotating sound heads, we can diagnose the absence of fetal movements with certainty. Finally, the A- and B-scan methods permit detection of the absence of growth of the biparietal diameter. This would obviously require a longer period of time (three examinations at weekly intervals). Needless to say, proving the absence of growth alone is not conclusive; this method must only be used together with the others mentioned above.

Radiographic examination can be dispensed with in clinical routine today; from the 20th to 30th week the detection of cranial signs by ultrasonics is distinctly superior to radiographic examination and of equal value later.

Abortions—Carneous Moles

(see Figs. 96–99, p. 130)

Ultrasonic diagnosis contributes little to the diagnosis of the various stages of abortion and is only a plaything in comparison to clinical examination and laboratory values. Ultrasonic diagnosis only acquires some significance as a useful supplementary method when a carneous mole is suspected, if it is a matter of shortening the duration of hospitalization with a qualitatively positive or semiquantitatively low chorion-gonadotropin value. Ultrasonic diagnosis is then used with the knowledge that even intact pregnancies can give low values.

In the case of the carneous mole, we find an embryonic sac that is mostly free of echos; only a few echos are caused by the trophoblasts, but the distinct reflections from the embryo are missing. It is an established fact that clinical practice differentiates between the incomplete and complete abortion according to whether the os uteri is open or has closed again. Ultrasonic diagnosis can give valuable indications if, as is occasionally observed, the cervical canal closes again without all parts of the embryo being totally ejected. For the sake of interest we illustrate such a case.

Breech Presentation

(see Figs. 100–106, p. 136)

Today it is considered extraordinarily important that prenatal diagnosis of breech presentation be certain. Some already argue that a primary section should be done in every case; this procedure, on the basis of our own investigations, is doubtless carried to excess. If external and rectal examination fail to give the desired results, and X-ray measurement of the pelvis, often performed at the same time, has not already clarified the situation with regard to the presenting part, we always use ultrasonic diagnosis. Often it will also be possible to dispense with radiographic diagnosis (radiographic pelvic measurement) altogether, if clinical palpation of the pelvis and ultrasonic measurement of the true conjugate makes the relationship of pelvis to head clear. Naturally, the biparietal diameter is measured at the same time.

Longitudinal section examination by the B-scan method permits reliable diagnosis of breech presentation, which is also superior to the X-ray picture in terms of money and time expenditure.

We show some interesting pictures of breech presentations in cases of malformation of the uterus. Besides this, other possible causes of breech presentation are hydramnios, abnormality of the upper aperture of the pelvis, and fetal malformations. It has been established that most breech presentations are observed in the 20th to 26th week of pregnancy and the final position has established itself by the 28th to 32th week. With the aid of ultra-sonic diagnosis, however, we have twice been able to record spontaneous turning immediately before and even at full term.

Malformations

(see Fig. 107, p. 144)

A communication received recently from STEIN *et al.* shows that US diagnosis of major fetal malformations yields valuable results. Anencephalus can be positively diagnosed. An example is presented in Fig. 107. Hydrocephalus can be diagnosed just as positively. Large omphalenteroceles, large meningomyeloceles as well as large cystic kidneys and ovarian tumors can be suspected.

Measuring the True Conjugate

(see Figs. 108–111, p. 147)

It is generally understood that because of the conventional external measurements of the pelvis only the internal dimensions of the small pelvis can be indicated. Pelvimetry plays a particulary important role in the case of breech presentation. With ultrasonic techniques in their present state, we must give preference, with regard to conclusiveness, to monoscopic or stereoscopic radiograph. Such radiography permits reliable assessment of all levels of the pelvis and also allows us to determine at a glance the shape of the pelvic duct, which in turn is of some significance for the progress of the birth and for comprehending the length of the anterior pelvic process. Disregarding a special technique that uses vaginal sound heads, we can say that only the routine use of ultrasonic diagnosis comes into consideration for the measurement of the true conjugate; the A-scan gives more accurate dimensions, but a check with the B-scan method should be carried out, in order to confirm that the shortest distance has actually been detected with the peaks of the A-scan. The sound head is applied on the symphysis and tilted in the direction of the promontorium; the patient's pelvis is slightly raised and the bladder is full.

The clinicaly important question arises of whether radiographic measurement of the pelvis can be replaced by ultrasonic diagnosis. Since we have used both methods in combination for 2 years, may we be permitted to make the following recommendation:

1. Whenever the true conjugate is measured by ultrasonics, palpation of the pelvis must be done by an experienced obstetrician, as the shape of the accessible sections of the sacrum and the mobility and shape of the coccygeal bone must be assessed. More important than the very difficult decision on the prominence of the spinae ischiadicae is the length of the sacro-spinal ligament. Here the free length of ligament between the tip of the spina and the edge of the sacrum should be an estimated two finger-widths.

2. In this way the head–pelvis ratio can be assessed safely in the great majority of cases, because the simultaneous measurement of the biparietal diameter, of course takes place in the same operation by ultrasonic means. Very rare exceptions are caused by the anthropoid pelvis. However, this is pointed out when the true conjugate is measured, if the distance is more than 12.5 cm. In such cases only antero–posterior X-ray measurement provides certainty.

We perform pelvimetry (ultrasonic and/or radiographic measurement) in the following cases:

1. Two of the three transverse external pelvic dimensions are shorter than the standard by more than 2 cm.

2. The conjugata externa is shorter than the standard by more than 1.5 cm (1 cm in case of breech presentation).

3. The history gives reason to suspect pelvic malformation (rickets, poliomyelitis, trauma, congenital dislocation of the hip-joint) or the Michaelis rhomboid gives indications of abnormalities.

4. Primiparae with movement of the head immediately before or at full term (unless the diagnosis of a placenta praevia is certain).

5. Undersize, with body length less than 150 cm.

Involution of the Uterus during the Puerperium

(see Figs. 112–115, p. 152)

On this subject we merely wish to show a few pictures for the sake of interest; they are intended to serve as practice in the detection of structures of the empty uterus and its surroundings. Clinically, ultrasonic diagnosis is not significance, since palpation gives quicker and equally reliable data.

Located between the symphysis and the navel, the part of the uterus above the symphysis after delivery of the placenta is 15 cm high and 10 to 12 cm wide. Because the contractions cease, the level of the navel is reached after two days; the level of the fundus then decreases by about a finger-width per day and on the 5th day it reaches about midway between the symphysis and navel. The boundary of the symphysis is reached on the 9th day. As we know, the speed of involution depends on various factors (weight of the child, hydramnios, infection, nutrition reflex), so that the range of variations is very great.

Ultrasonic Diagnosis in Gynecology

(see Figs. 116 127, p. 158)

In a clinical hospital, gynecological ultrasonic diagnosis can never have the same importance ascribed to it as it does in the obstetric field. To avoid any misunderstandings, we would like to remark, that we hold as a guiding principle, now as before, that examination by inspection and, above all, palpation by practiced hands cannot be replaced by any other primary method. Only in cases of pronounced obesity and tumors of the ovaries and Fallopian tubes in high positions, can ultrasonic diagnosis make a decisive contribution, if examination under anesthesia is not desired in its place. Whether the preoperative uncertainty that occurs in a few cases, be it a large myoma or an ovarian tumor, has to be solved in a sense of diagnostic perfectionism before the laparotomy, is a matter of judgement. It is in fact possible to carry out this differential diagnosis satisfactorily with ultrasonics and at the same time draw interesting conclusions on the nature of ovarian tumors.

The *ovarian cyst* is characterized by good sound conduction, the posterior wall of the tumor also shows up well under low intensity and without depth compensation. If the cyst is unilocular, the inner space appears as an echo-free homogeneous image, and the sactosalpinx behaves similarly. With the multilocular cyst, distinct echos, which are reflected from the chamber walls, are to be seen within larger echo-free regions.

Myomata, especially solid nodules, have poor sound conduction, making greater depth compensation necessary for determining the posterior boundary. It is difficult to differentiate between *solid ovarian tumors* and myomata, particularly softened nodules.

Pregnancy with Uterine Myoma

(see Figs. 128–130, p. 174)

The clinical practitioner should not mistake a uterine myoma for pregnancy or vice versa. Nevertheless, such cases are continually reported, especially if a pregnant patient mentions menstruation-like hemorrhages in her history. In all cases of doubt, ultrasonic diagnosis provides clarification with the use of the B-scan, Doppler, or M-scan methods. With regard to combining these three methods with the endocrine parameters, see page 3.

Ultrasonic diagnosis can be used effectively if both pregnancy and a uterine myoma are present. Above all, the extent of cervical or isthmic subserosal myomal nodules or intraligamentary myomata can be determined, if the patient is observed only in an advanced state of pregnancy. The findings are pertinent to the conduct of the birth, if, with insertion on the posterior or lateral wall, the question of an obstacle to delivery exists. Reliable prognoses however, can only be made in a few cases. When uterine myoma and pregnancy are combined, neither the ability to carry the pregnancy to full term, nor the luxation of the tumor out of the small pelvis during the period of opening, are predictable.

Ultrasonic Diagnosis on the Upper Abdomen

(see Figs. 131–138, p. 178)

We lack personal experience in detecting tumors of the pancreas and spleen. However, with the following pictures we report a few typical findings from examinations of the liver and kidneys, to demonstrate that the examination gives useful results by simple means.

The kidneys are best examined with the patient in the prone position. Using the B-scan method, a sub-costal cross section and a bilateral-paravertebral longitudinal section are carried out. Ultrasonic diagnosis cannot compete with differentiated radiographic examination in regard to accuracy; yet it does assume a role in routine work, if the site of a planned kidney biopsy has to be determined.

The liver is shown as a homogenous, echofree organ; examination is carried out in the dorsal position. In the case of cirrhosis and metastasis, multiple reflections can be seen.

Evidence of Early Pregnancy

Nachweis einer Frühschwangerschaft
Mise en évidence d'une grossesse au stade précoce
Diagnóstico del embarazo precoz
Determinazione della gravidanza in uno stadio precoce

Fig. 1. Normal Pregnancy in the 7th Week

Cross section above the symphysis with an amenorrhoea of 7 weeks.
The embryo can be seen inside the uterine cavity.
Scale graduation: 2 cm per square. Sound frequency: 2 MHz

Abb. 1. Intakte Schwangerschaft in der 7. Woche

Querschnitt oberhalb der Symphyse bei einer Amenorrhoe von 7 Wochen.
Innerhalb der Fruchthöhle ist die Frucht zu erkennen. Skaleneinteilung pro Feld 2 cm. Schallfrequenz 2 MHZ

Fig. 1. Grossesse intacte dans la 7ᵉ semaine

Coupe transversale au-dessus de la symphyse avec aménorrhée de 7 semaines.
On perçoit le foetus à l'intérieur de la cavité amniotique. Graduation par champ 2 cm. Fréquence de son 2 MHz

Fig. 1. Embarazo normal en la séptima semana de gestación

Corte transversal suprapúbico en una paciente con amenorrea de 7 semanas.
En la cavidad amniótica pueden observarse estructuras fetales. 1 división de escala=2 cm. Frecuencia del ultrasonido=2 Mega Hertz (MHz)

Fig. 1. Gravidanza intatta nella settima settimana

Sezione trasversale al di sopra della sinfisi con amenorrea di sette settimane.
E' possibile osservare il feto all'interno del cavo amniotico. Graduazione per campo 2 cm. Frequenza 2 MHZ

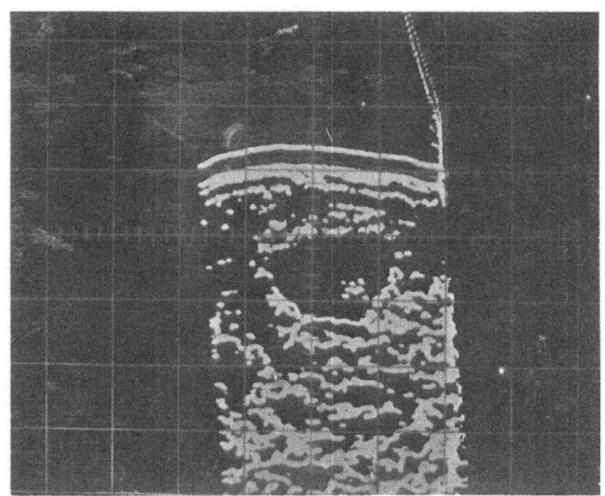

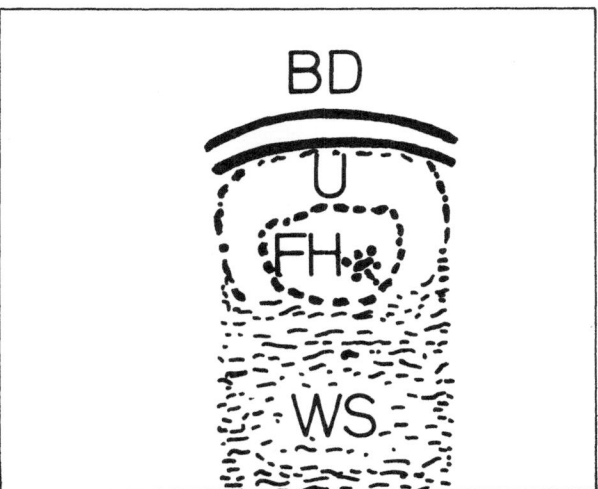

1

Determining the Biparietal Diameter

Bestimmung des biparietalen Durchmessers
Détermination du diamètre bipariétal
Determinación del diámetro biparietal
Determinazione del diametro biparietale

Fig. 2. Pregnancy at Full Term

Suprapubic cross section used in measuring the
the biparietal diameter with B-scan.
Complete circumference of cranium with central
echo, biparietal diameter: 9 cm. Scale graduation: 2 cm/square

Fig. 3. Pregnancy at Full Term

Measurement of the biparietal diameter with A-
scan (Amplitude diagram); same case as
Fig. 2.
ME is exactly central between B_1 and B_2. The
distance from B_1 to B_2 corresponds to the biparietal diameter

Abb. 2. Gravidität am Termin

Suprasymphysärer Querschnitt für die Messung
des biparietalen Durchmessers mit B-Bild.
Ganzer Schädelumfang mit Mittelecho, biparietaler Durchmesser von 9 cm. Skaleneinteilung
pro Feld 2 cm

Abb. 3. Gravidität am Termin

Messung des biparietalen Durchmessers mit A-
Bild (Amplitudenbild), gleicher Fall wie
Abb. 2.
ME ist genau zwischen B_1 und B_2. Die Entfer-
nung von B_1 und B_2 entspricht dem biparietalen
DM

Fig. 2. Grossesse au terme

Coupe transversale suprasymphysaire pour le
mesurage du diamètre bipariétal par image B.
Circonférence de crâne complète avec écho médian, diamètre bipariétal de 9 cm. Graduation
par champ 2 cm

Fig. 3. Grossesse au terme

Mesurage du diamètre bipariétal par image A
(image à amplitudes), même cas que l'image 2.
ME se trouve exactement entre B_1 et B_2. La
distance entre B_1 et B_2 correspond au diamètre
bipariétal

Fig. 2. Embarazo a término

Corte transversal suprapúbico para la medición
del diámetro biparietal con imagen B.
Se puede observar un corte de la cabeza fetal
con eco medio. Diámetro biparietal = 9,0 cm. 1
división de escala   2 cm

Fig. 3. Embarazo a término

Mismo caso de la figura 2. Medición del
diámetro biparietal con el sistema A.
El eco medio se encuentra a igual distancia entre
B 1 y B 2. La distancia B 1 a B 2 corresponde
al diámetro biparietal

Fig. 2. Gravidanza a termine

Sezione al di sopra della sinfisi per la misurazione del diametro biparietale con l'immagine B.
Circonferenza completa del cranio con eco mediano, diametro biparietale di 9 cm. Graduazione per campo 2 cm

Fig. 3. Gravidanza a termine

Misurazione del diametro biparietale con l'immagine A (Immagine di amplitudine), caso
uguale a quello della figura 2.
ME si trova esattamente fra B_1 e B_2. La distanza
fra B_1 e B_2 corrisponde al diametro biparietale

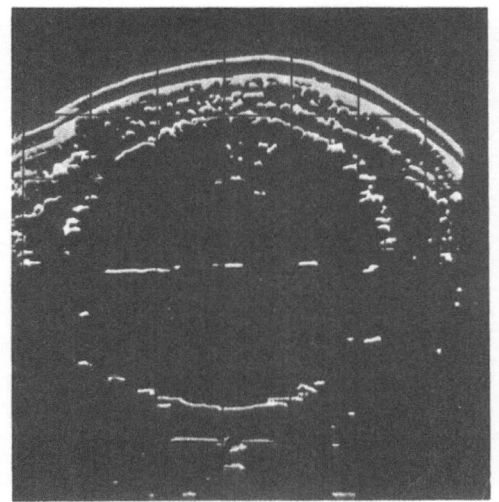
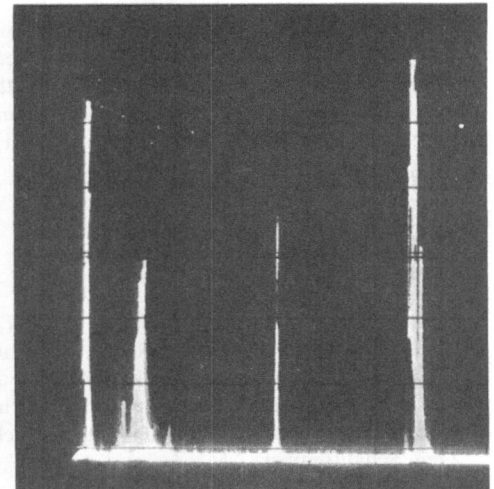

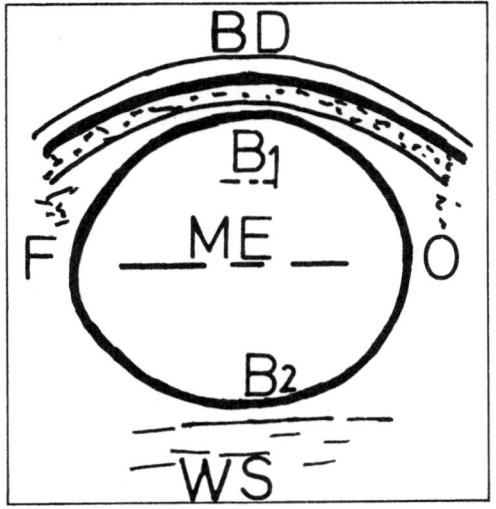

BD

B₁

ME

F   O

B₂

WS

2

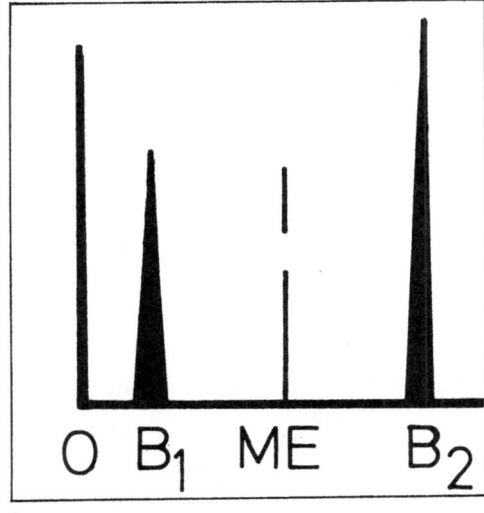

O   B₁   ME   B₂

3

Fig. 4. Pregnancy at Full Term

Cross section of a fetal thorax in the 38th week of pregnancy; same case as Fig. 3. Above the torso, the placenta can be seen. Scale graduation: 2 cm per square. Sound frequency: 2 MHz

Abb. 4. Gravidität am Termin

Querschnitt eines kindlichen Thorax bei einer Schwangerschaft in der 38. Woche, gleicher Fall wie Abb. 3. Oberhalb des Rumpfes ist die Plazenta zu erkennen. Skaleneinteilung pro Feld 2 cm. Schallfrequenz 2 MHZ

Fig. 4. Grossesse au terme

Coupe transversale du thorax d'un enfant dans la 38ᵉ semaine d'une grossesse, même cas que l'image 3. Audessus du tronc on aperçoit le placenta. Graduation par champ 2 cm. Fréquence de son 2 MHz

Fig. 4. Embarazo a término

Mismo caso de la figura 3. Corte transversal por el tórax fetal con imagen B. 38 semanas de gestación. Sobre el cuerpo fetal se puede observar la placenta. 1 división de escala = 2 cm. Frecuencia de ultrasonido = 2 MHz

Fig. 4. Gravidanza a termine

Sezione del torace del feto nella 38a settimana di gravidanza. Caso uguale a quello della figura 3. Sopra il tronco si osserva la placenta. Graduazione per campo 2 cm. Frequenza 2 MHZ

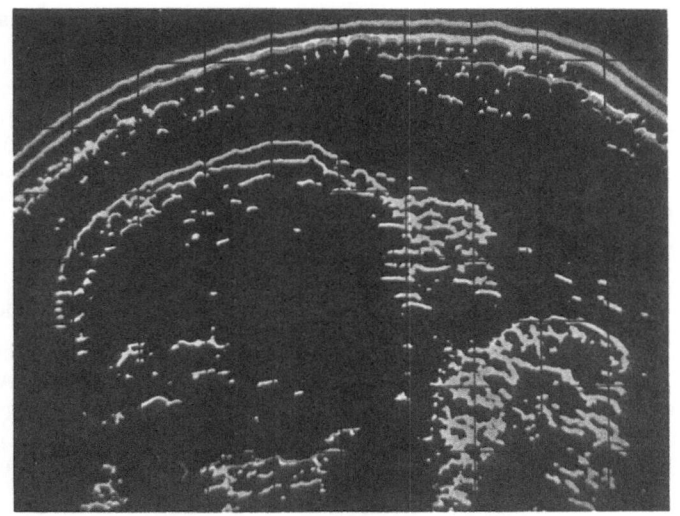

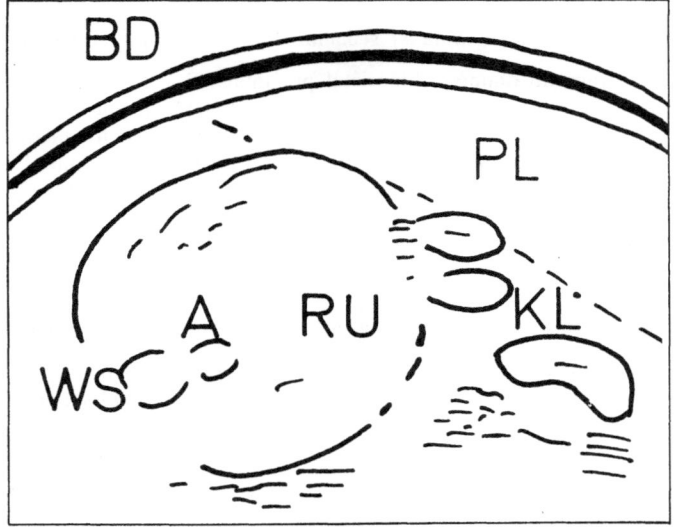

4

Fig. 5. Pregnancy in the 30th Week

Measurement of the biparietal diameter with B-scan in a pregnancy in the 30th week. Central echo. Lateral reflection can be seen above the central echo

Fig. 6. Pregnancy in the 30th Week

Measurement of the biparietal diameter with A-scan; same case as Fig. 5.
Here, the central echo also lies between the initial and final echos. After the final echo, the echo of the promontorium appears

Abb. 5. Gravidität in der 30. Woche

Messung des biparietalen DM mit B-Bild bei einer Schwangerschaft in der 30. Woche. Mittelecho, oberhalb der Mittelechos sind Lateralreflexionen zu erkennen

Abb. 6. Gravidität in der 30. Woche

Messung des biparietalen DM mit A-Bild, gleicher Fall wie Abb. 5.
Mittelecho liegt hier ebenfalls zwischen Initial- und Endecho. Nach dem Endecho erscheint das Echo des Promontorium

Fig. 5. Grossesse dans la 30ᵉ semaine

Mesurage du diamètre bipariétal par image B dans la 30ᵉ semaine d'une grossesse. Echo médian. On aperçoit des réflexions latérales au-dessus de l'écho médian

Fig. 6. Grossesse dans la 30ᵉ semaine

Mesurage du diamètre bipariétal par image A, même cas que l'image 5.
L'écho médian se trouve ici également entre l'écho initial et l'écho final. Après l'écho final apparaît l'écho du promontoire

Fig. 5. Embarazo de 30 semanas de gestación

Medición del diámetro biparietal con imagen. B. Sobre el eco medio pueden observarse reflexiones laterales

Fig. 6. Embarazo de 30 semanas de gestación

Medición del diámetro biparietal con imagen A. Mismo caso de la figura 5.
El eco medio se encuentra entre el eco inicial y el final. Detras del eco final se observa el eco del promontorio

Fig. 5. Trentesima settimana di gravidanza

Misurazione del diametro biparietale con l'immagine B nella trentesima settimana di gravidanza. Eco mediano, sopra il quale si osservano riflessi laterali

Fig. 6. Trentesima settimana di gravidanza

Misurazione del diametro biparietale con l'immagine A, caso uguale a quello della figura 5.
Anche qui l'eco mediano è situato fra l'eco iniziale e l'eco finale. Dopo l'eco finale appare l'eco del promontorio

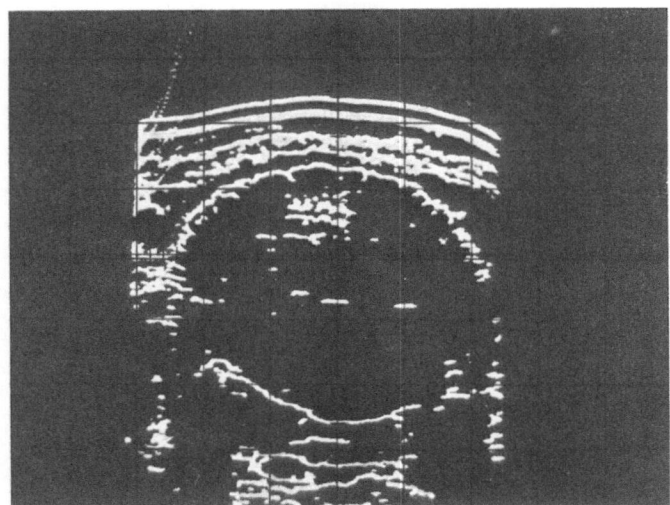

5

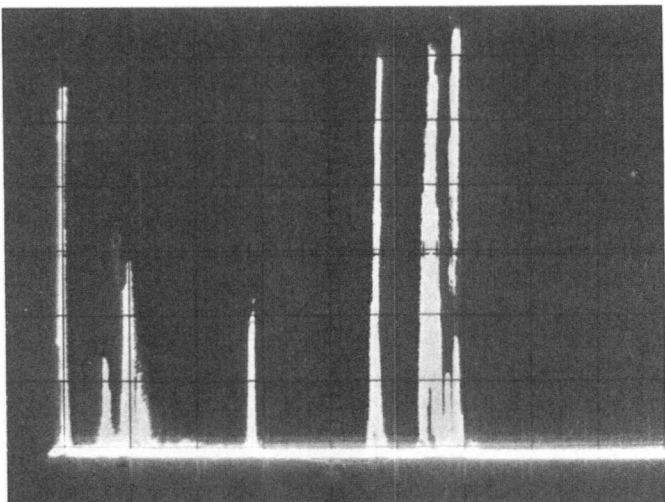

6

Fig. 7. Pregnancy in the 30th Week

Child's thorax in cross section; same case as above.
Small members are clearly visible beside the thorax

Abb. 7. Gravidität in der 30. Woche

Kindlicher Thorax im Querschnitt, gleicher Fall wie oben.
Neben Thorax sind deutlich kleine Teile zu sehen

Fig. 7. Grossesse dans la 30ᵉ semaine

Thorax d'enfant en coupe transversale, même cas que ci-dessus.
A côté du thorax on aperçoit nettement des parties foetales

Fig. 7. Embarazo de 30 semanas de gestación

Corte transversal de tórax fetal. Imagen B.
Mismo caso de la figura 6.
Al lado del tórax pueden observarse extremidades fetales

Fig. 7. Trentesima settimana di gravidanza

Torace del feto in sezione, caso uguale a quello della figura precedente.
Accanto al torace sono visibili altre parti del feto

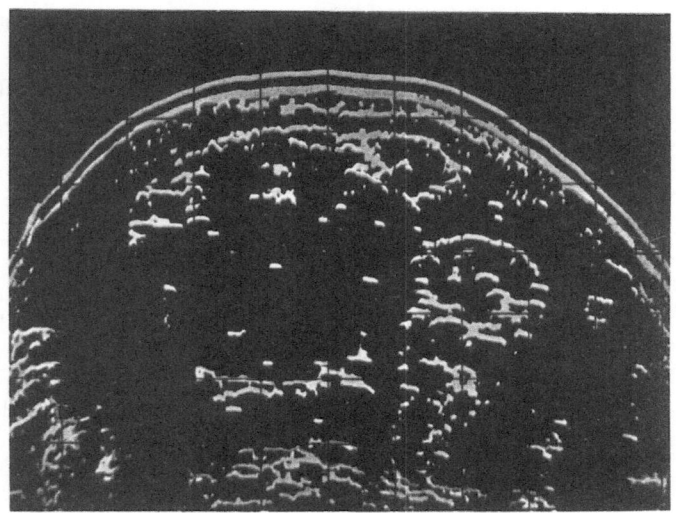

7

Fig. 8. Pregnancy in the 40th Week

Cross section above the symphysis at location of cranium. Biparietal diameter with B-diagram: 9.6 cm. Complete circumference of cranium, central echo. Lateral reflections are visible above the central echo

Fig. 9. Pregnancy in the 40th Week

Same case as Fig. 8, biparietal diameter with A-scan (amplitude diagram) is also 9.6 cm. Central echo between initial and final echos

Abb. 8. Schwangerschaft in der 40. Woche

Querschnitt oberhalb der Symphyse bei Schädellage. Biparietaler DM mit B-Bild 9,6 cm. Ganzer Schädelumfang, Mittelecho, oberhalb der Mittelechos sind Lateralreflexionen sichtbar

Abb. 9. Schwangerschaft in der 40. Woche

Gleicher Fall wie Abb. 8, biparietaler DM mit A-Bild (Amplituden-Bild) beträgt ebenfalls 9,6 cm. Mittelecho zwischen Initial- und Endecho

Fig. 8. Grossesse dans la 40ᵉ semaine

Coupe transversale au-dessus de la symphyse, avec présentation du sommet. Diamètre bipariétal par image B 9,6 cm. Circonférence de crâne complète, écho médian, on aperçoit des réflexions latérales au-dessus de l'écho médian

Fig. 9. Grossesse dans la 40ᵉ semaine

Même cas que l'image 8, le diamètre bipariétal par image A (image à amplitudes) mesure également 9,6 cm. Echo médian entre l'écho initial et l'écho final

Fig. 8. Embarazo a término-40 semanas de gestación

Corte transversal suprapúbico con representación de la cabeza fetal. Diámetro biparietal con imagen B: 9,6 cm. En el corte de la cabeza fetal se puede observar el eco medio, sobre el cual se encuentran reflejos laterales

Fig. 9. Embarazo a término-40 semanas de gestación

Mismo caso de la figura anterior. Medición del diámetro biparietal con imagen A: 9,6 cm. El eco medio se encuentra entre el eco inicial y el eco final

Fig. 8. Quarantesima settimana di gravidanza

Sezione al di sopra della sinfisi, con presentazione craniale. Diametro biparietale con immagine B: 9,6 cm. Circonferenza completa del cranio, eco mediano, al di sopra del quale si osservano riflessi laterali

Fig. 9. Quarantesima settimana di gravidanza

Caso uguale a quello della figura 8, diametro biparietale con immagine A (immagine di amplitudine) parimenti uguale a 9,6 cm. Eco mediano fra l'eco iniziale e l'eco finale

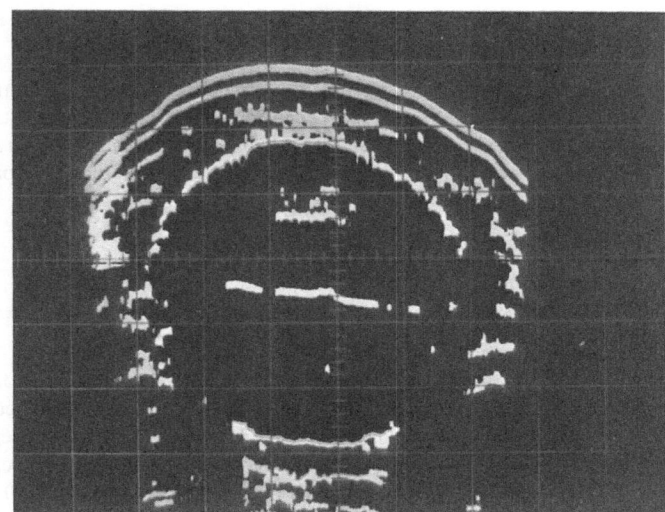

8

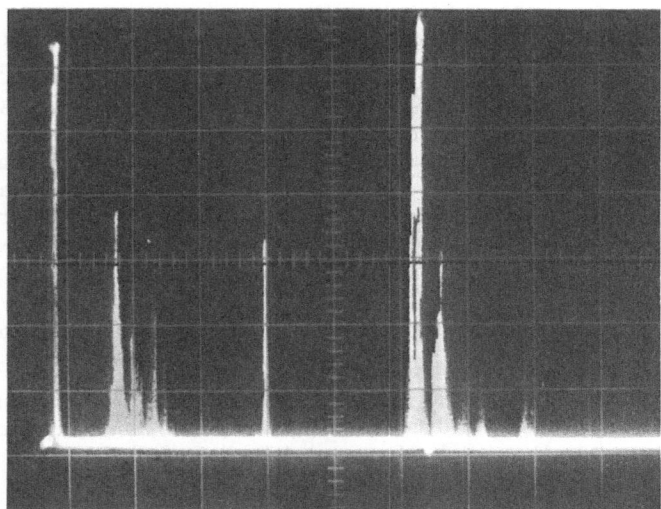

9

Fig. 10. Falx cerebri in the Transverse Diameter

Cross section above the symphysis in a pregnancy in the 30th week, falx cerebri (central echo) in the transverse diameter. Biparietal diameter is 7.8 cm; sides of squares are 1 cm

Fig. 11. Falx cerebri almost in In-Line Diameter

Cross section above the symphysis, slightly above the entrance to the pelvis. Here the falx cerebri (central echo) is almost in line (upright position). Biparietal diameter is 10 cm

Abb. 10. Falx cerebri im queren Durchmesser

Suprasymphysärer Querschnitt bei einer Gravidität in der 30. Woche, Falx cerebri (Mittelecho) im queren Durchmesser. Biparietaler Durchmesser beträgt 7,8 cm. Kantenlänge pro Feld 1 cm

Abb. 11. Falx cerebri fast im geraden Durchmesser

Querschnitt oberhalb der Symphyse, also etwas über dem Beckeneingang. Hier steht die Falx cerebri (Mittelecho) fast im geraden Durchmesser.(Hoher Geradstand). Biparietaler Durchmesser beträgt 10 cm

Fig. 10. Faux du cerveau en diamètre transversal

Coupe transversale suprasymphysaire dans la 30e semaine d'une grossesse, faux du cerveau (écho médian) en son diamètre transversal. Le diamètre bipariétal mesure 7,8 cm. Longueur de côté par champ 1 cm

Fig. 11. Faux du cerveau quasi en diamètre perpendiculaire

Coupe transversale au-dessus de la symphyse, donc un peu au-dessus du détroit supérieur du bassin. La faux du cerveau (écho médian) se trouve ici quasi en son diamètre perpendiculaire (position droite prononcée). Le diamètre bipariétal mesure 10 cm

Fig. 10. La hoz cerebral en diámetro transverso

Corte transversal suprapúbico, imagen B. Embarazo de 30 semanas de gestación. El eco medio representa la hoz en diámetro transverso. El diámetro biparietal es de 7,8 cm. 1 división de escala = 1 cm

Fig. 11. La hoz cerebral en diámetro antero-posterior

Corte transversal suprapúbico, imagen B. El eco medio representa la hoz en diámetro antero-posterior. Diámetro biparietal: 10 cm

Fig. 10. Falce del cervello in diametro trasversale

Sezione sopra la sinfisi nella trentesima settimana di gravidanza, falce del cervello (eco mediano) in diametro trasversale. Il diametro biparietale è di 7,8 cm. Lunghezza del lato per campo 1 cm

Fig. 11. Falce del cervello quasi in diametro perpendicolare

Sezione sopra la sinfisi, ossia leggermente al di sopra dello stretto superiore del bacino. La falce del cervello (eco mediano) si trova quasi nel diametro perpendicolare (posizione eretta pronunciata). Il diametro biparietale è di 10 cm

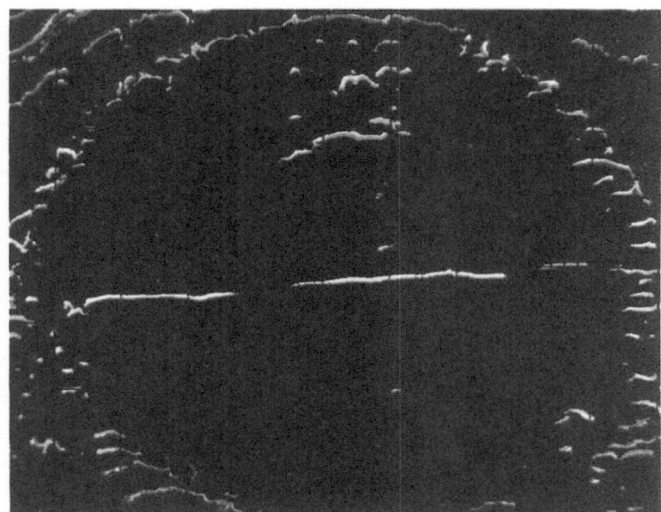

10

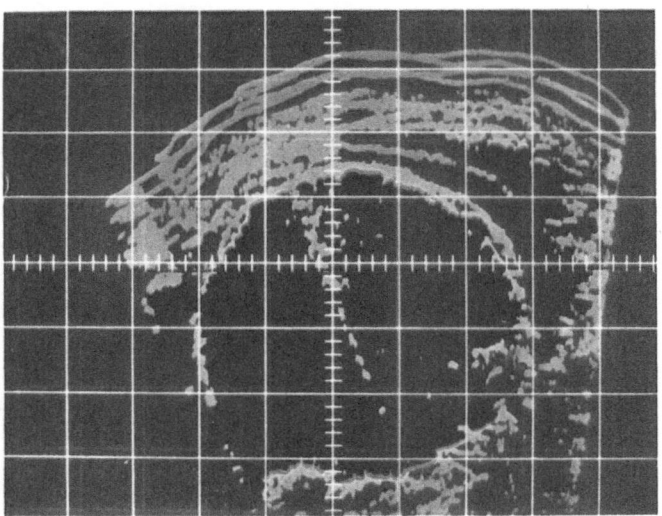

11

Monitoring Fetal Growth

Verfolgung des fetalen Wachstums
Observation de la croissance foetale
Observación del crecimiento fetal
Osservazione della crescita del feto

Fig. 12.   7th Week of Pregnancy
Fig. 13.   9th Week of Pregnancy
Fig. 14. 11th Week of Pregnancy

Abb. 12.   7. Schwangerschaftswoche
Abb. 13.   9. Schwangerschaftswoche
Abb. 14. 11. Schwangerschaftswoche

Fig. 12.   7^e semaine de grossesse
Fig. 13.   9^e semaine de grossesse
Fig. 14. 11^e semaine de grossesse

Fig. 12.   7 semanas de gestación
Fig. 13.   9 semanas de gestación
Fig. 14. 11 semanas de gestación

Fig. 12.   7a settimana di gravidanza
Fig. 13.   9a settimana di gravidanza
Fig. 14. 11a settimana di gravidanza

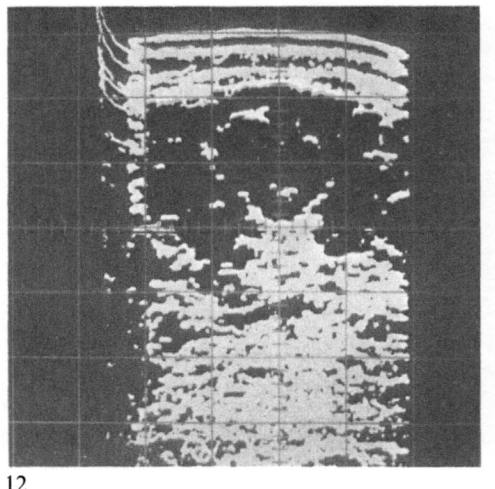

12

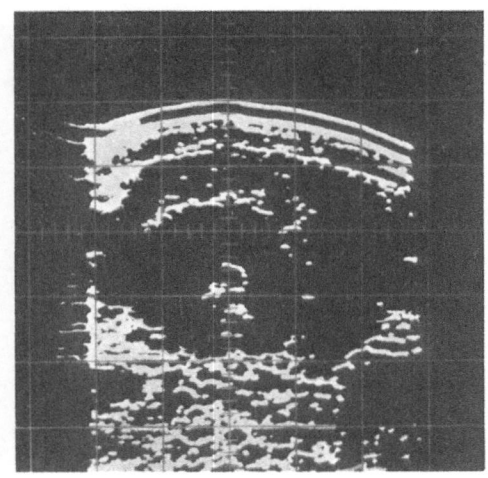

13

14

Fig. 15. 13th Week of Pregnancy

Fig. 16. 15th Week of Pregnancy

Fig. 17. 17th Week of Pregnancy

Fig. 18. 18th Week of Pregnancy

Fig. 19. 20th Week of Pregnancy

Fig. 20. 22nd Week of Pregnancy

Abb. 15. 13. Schwangerschaftswoche

Abb. 16. 15. Schwangerschaftswoche

Abb. 17. 17. Schwangerschaftswoche

Abb. 18. 18. Schwangerschaftswoche

Abb. 19. 20. Schwangerschaftswoche

Abb. 20. 22. Schwangerschaftswoche

Fig. 15. 13^e semaine de grossesse

Fig. 16. 15^e semaine de grossesse

Fig. 17. 17^e semaine de grossesse

Fig. 18. 18^e semaine de grossesse

Fig. 19. 20^e semaine de grossesse

Fig. 20. 22^e semaine de grossesse

Fig. 15. 13 semanas de gestación

Fig. 16. 15 semanas de gestación

Fig. 17. 17 semanas de gestación

Fig. 18. 18 semanas de gestación

Fig. 19. 20 semanas de gestación

Fig. 20. 22 semanas de gestación

Fig. 15. 13a settimana di gravidanza

Fig. 16. 15a settimana di gravidanza

Fig. 17. 17a settimana di gravidanza

Fig. 18. 18a settimana di gravidanza

Fig. 19. 20a settimana di gravidanza

Fig. 20. 22a settimana di gravidanza

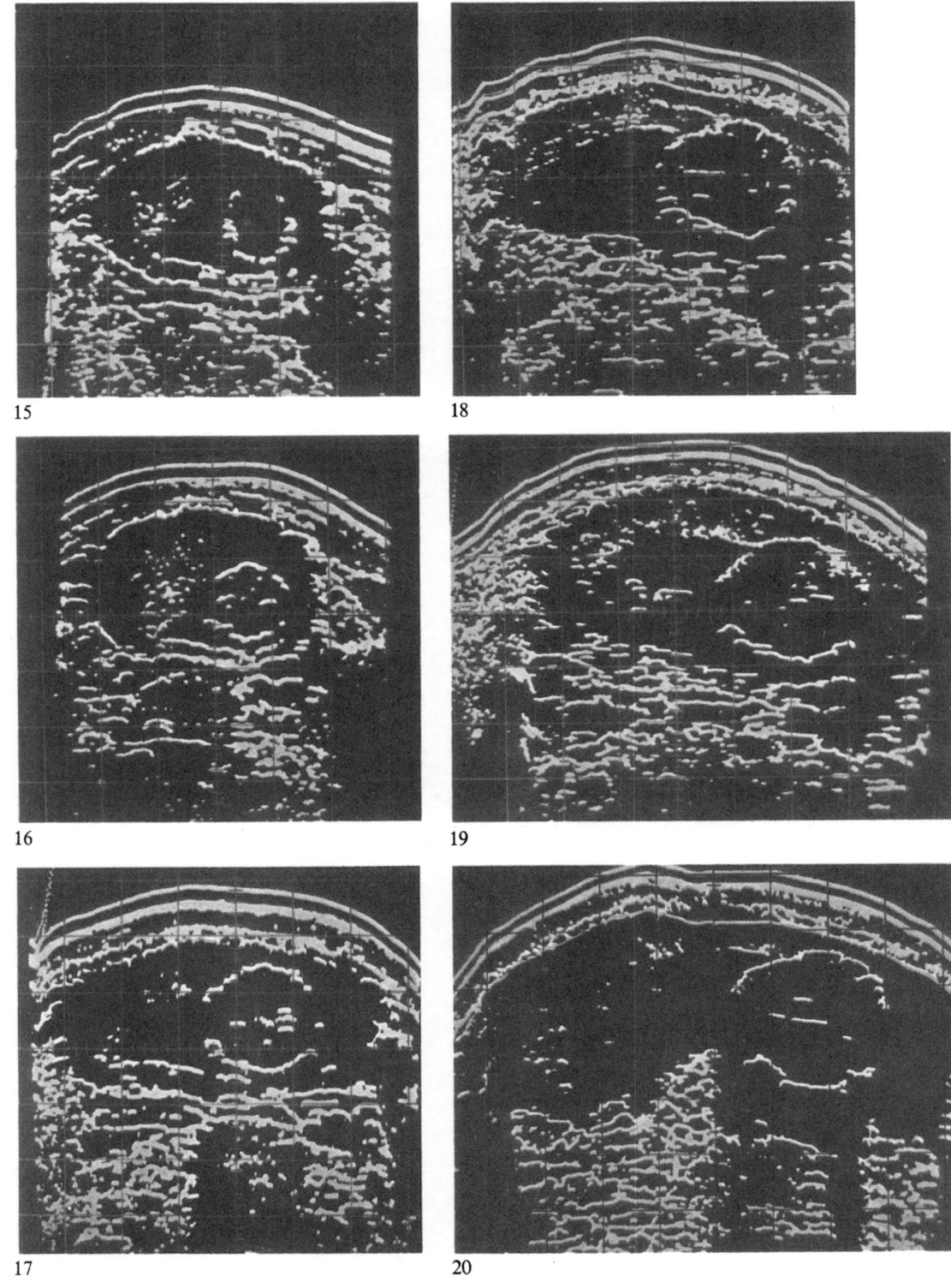

15

16

17

18

19

20

Fig. 21. 24th Week of Pregnancy
Fig. 22. 26th Week of Pregnancy
Fig. 23. 28th Week of Pregnancy

Abb. 21. 24. Schwangerschaftswoche
Abb. 22. 26. Schwangerschaftswoche
Abb. 23. 28. Schwangerschaftswoche

Fig. 21. 24ᵉ semaine de grossesse
Fig. 22. 26ᵉ semaine de grossesse
Fig. 23. 28ᵉ semaine de grossesse

Fig. 21. 24 semanas de gestación
Fig. 22. 26 semanas de gestación
Fig. 23. 28 semanas de gestación

Fig. 21. 24a settimana di gravidanza
Fig. 22. 26a settimana di gravidanza
Fig. 23. 28a settimana di gravidanza

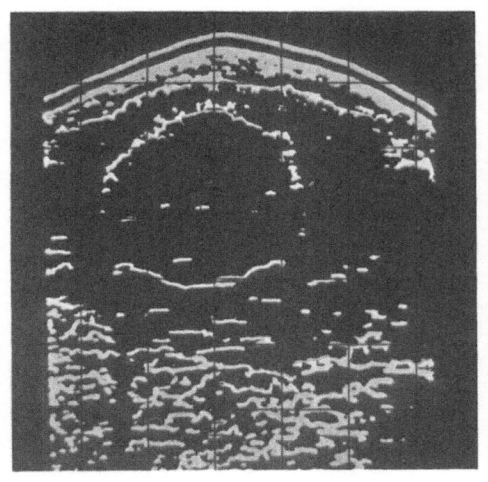

21

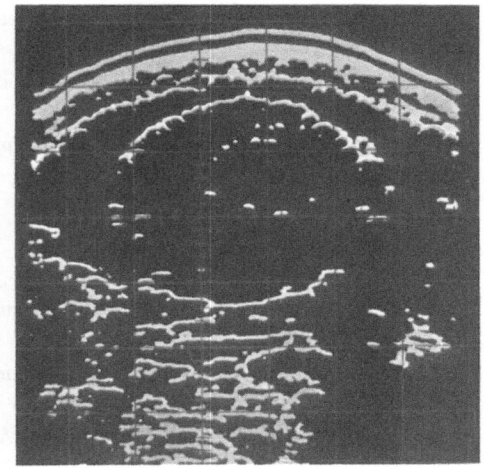

22

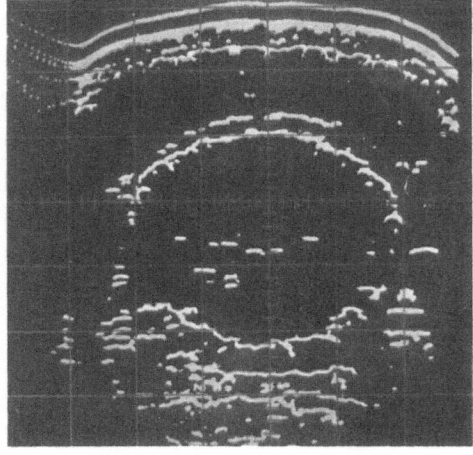

23

Fig. 24. 30th Week of Pregnancy, Measurement with A- and B-Scans

Fig. 25. 34th Week of Pregnancy, Measurement with A- and B-Scans

Fig. 26. Child's Head at Full Term with A- and B-Scans

Abb. 24. 30. Schwangerschaftswoche, Messung mit A- und B-Bild

Abb. 25. 34. Schwangerschaftswoche, Messung mit A- und B-Bild

Abb. 26. Kindlicher Kopf am Termin mit A- und B-Bild

Fig. 24. 30ᵉ semaine de grossesse, mesurage par images A et B

Fig. 25. 34ᵉ semaine de grossesse, mesurage par images A et B

Fig. 26. Tête d'enfant au terme, par images A et B

Fig. 24. Embarazo de 30 semanas. Imagen B y A

Fig. 25. Embarazo de 34 semanas. Imagen B y A

Fig. 26. Cabeza fetal en embarazo a término. Imagen B y A

Fig. 24. 30a settimana di gravidanza, misurazione con l'immagine A e B

Fig. 25. 34a settimana di gravidanza, misurazione con l'immagine A e B

Fig. 26. Testa del bambino al termine della gravidanza con l'immagine A e B

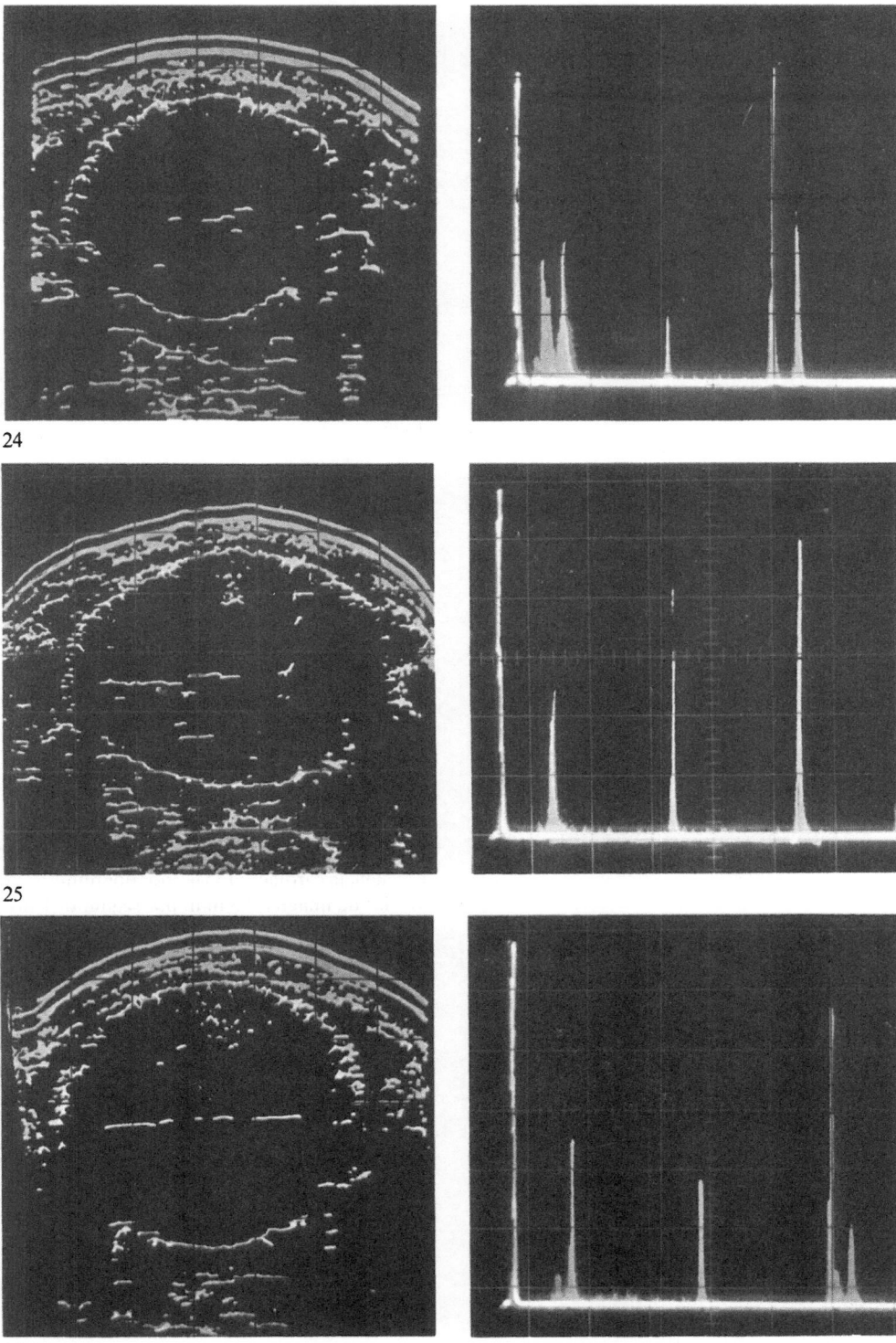

24

25

26

Detection of the Fetal Heart Action

Nachweis der fetalen Herzaktion
Mise en évidence de l'activité cardiaque
Demonstración de la actividad cardíaca fetal
Rivelazione dell'attività cardiaca del feto

Fig. 27. Fetal Heart Action in the 30th Week (M-Method)

Intra-uterine recording of fetal heart movement in the 30th week: 135/min. Chart speed is 25 mm/sec. Scale graduations are 1 cm/sections

Abb. 27. Fetale Herzaktion in der 30. Woche (M-Methode)

Intrauterin registrierte fetale Herzbewegung in der 30. Woche, 135/min. Laufgeschwindigkeit beträgt 25 mm/sec. Skaleneinteilung pro Feld 1 cm

Fig. 27. Activité cardiaque foetale dans la 30ᵉ semaine (méthode M)

Enregistrement intra-utérin d'un mouvement cardiaque foetal dans la 30ᵉ semaine, 135/min. La vitesse de marche est de 25 mm/sec. Graduation par champ 1 cm

Fig. 27. Actividad cardiaca fetal — 30 semanas de gestación (Sistema M)

Frecuencia cardiaca: 135 latidos por minuto. Velocidas de imagen: 25 mm. por segundo. 1 división de escala = 1 cm

Fig. 27. Attività cardiaca fetale nella 30a settimana di gravidanza (metodo M)

Registrazione intrauterina di un movimento cardiaco fetale nella 30a settimana, 135/min. La velocità di avanzamento è di 25 mm/sec, la graduazione per campo 1 cm

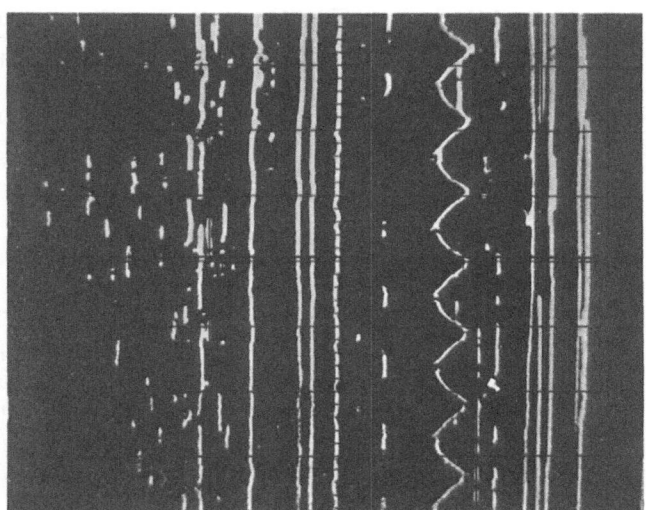

27

Fig. 28. Fetal Heart Action in the 30th Week (M-Method)

Same case as Fig. 27; heart action also 135/min. Scale divisions here are 0.5 cm

Fig. 29. Fetal Heart Movement in the 32nd Week

Recording of fetal heart action by the M-method. Chart speed: 5 mm/sec. Scale divisions: 3 cm/section. Fetal heart rate: 134/min

Abb. 28. Fetale Herzaktion in der 30. Woche (M-Methode)

Gleicher Fall wie Abb. 27. Herzaktion beträgt ebenfalls 135/min. Skaleneinteilung beträgt hier 0,5 cm

Abb. 29. Fetale Herzbewegung in der 32. Woche

Registrierung der fetalen Herzaktion mit M-Methode. Laufgeschwindigkeit: 5 mm/sec. Skaleneinteilung pro Feld 3 cm. Fetale Herzfrequenz: 134/min

Fig. 28. Activité cardiaque foetale dans la 30ᵉ semaine (méthode M)

Même cas que l'image 27, l'activité cardiaque est également de 135/min. La graduation est ici de 0,5 cm

Fig. 29. Mouvement cardiaque foetal dans la 32ᵉ semaine

Enregistrement de l'activité cardiaque foetal par la méthode M. Vitesse de marche: 5 mm/sec. Graduation par champ 3 cm. Fréquence cardiaque foetale: 134/min

Fig. 28. Actividad cardiaca fetal — 30 semanas de gestación (Sistema M)

Mismo caso de la figura anterior. Frecuencia cardiaca: 135 latidos por minuto. 1 división de escala = 0,5 cm

Fig. 29. Actividad cardiaca fetal — 32 semanas de gestación

Sistema M. Frecuencia cardiaca: 134 latidos por minuto. Velocidad de imagen: 5 mm por segundo. 1 división de escala = 3 cm

Fig. 28. Attività cardiaca fetale nella 30a settimana (metodo M)

Caso uguale a quello della figura 27. L'attività cardiaca è parimenti di 135/min. La graduazione è di 0,5 cm

Fig. 29. Movimento cadiaco fetale nella 32a settimana

Registrazione dell'attività cardiaca fetale con il metodo M. Velocità di avanzamento 5 mm/sec. Graduazione per campo 3 cm. Frequenza cardiaca fetale 134/min

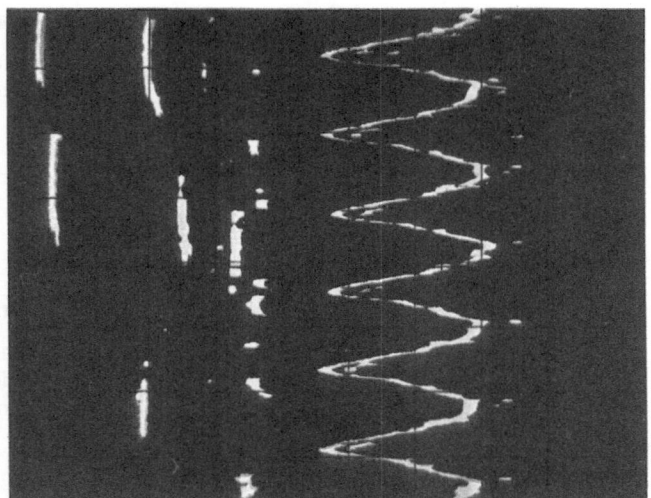

28

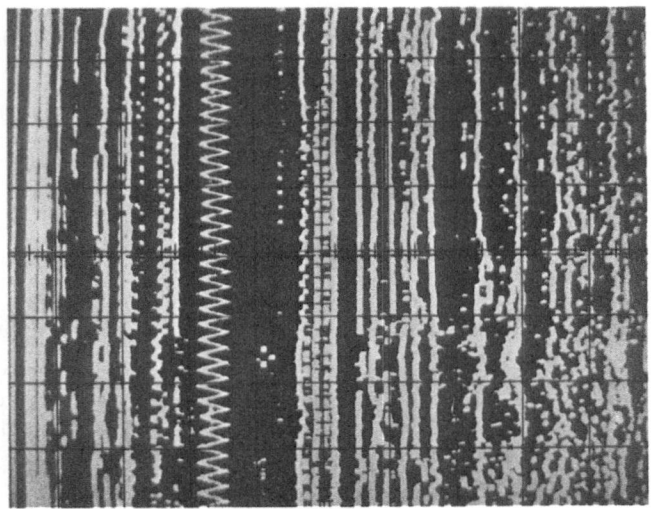

29

Fig. 30. Fetal Heart Action in the 34th Weeks

Intra-uterine recording of fetal heart action: 135/min. Chart speed: 25 mm/sec. Scale divisions: 2 cm

Fig. 31. Fetal Heart Action in the 34th Week

Same case as Fig. 30, with scale divisions of 1 cm/section. Chart speed: 25 mm/sec

Abb. 30. Fetale Herzaktion in der 34. Woche

Intrauterin registrierte Herzaktion des Fetus, 135/min. Laufgeschwindigkeit: 25 mm/sec. Skaleneinteilung 2 cm

Abb. 31. Fetale Herzaktion in der 34. Woche

Gleicher Fall wie Abb. 30, jedoch beträgt die Skaleneinteilung pro Feld 1 cm. Laufgeschwindigkeit: 25 mm/sec

Fig. 30. Activité cardiaque foetale dans la 34ᵉ semaine

Enregistrement intra-utérin de l'activité cardiaque du foetus, 135/min. Vitesse de marche: 25 mm/sec. Graduation 2 cm

Fig. 31. Activité cardiaque foetale dans la 34ᵉ semaine

Même cas que l'image 30, mais la graduation par champ mesure 1 cm. Vitesse de marche: 25 mm/sec

Fig. 30. Actividad cardiaca fetal — 34 semanas de gestación

Frecuencia cardiaca: 135 latidos por minuto. Velocidad de imagen: 25 mm por segundo. 1 división de escala = 2 cm

Fig. 31. Actividad cardiaca fetal

Mismo caso de la figura anterior. 1 división de escala = 1 cm. Velocidad de imagen: 25 mm por segundo.

Fig. 30. Attività cardiaca fetale nella 34a settimana

Registrazione intrauterina dell'attività cardiaca del feto, 135/min. Velocità di avanzamento: 25 mm/sec. Graduazione 2 cm

Fig. 31. Attività cardiaca fetale nella 34a settimana

Caso uguale a quello della fig. 30, ma la graduazione per campo è di 1 cm. Velocità di avanzamento: 25 mm/sec

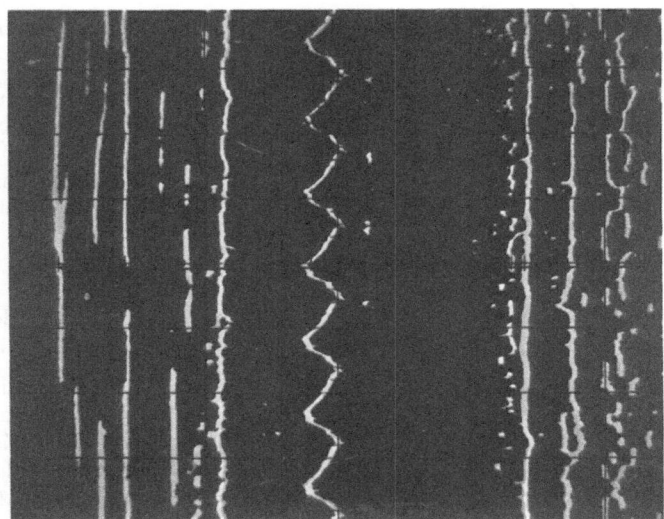

30

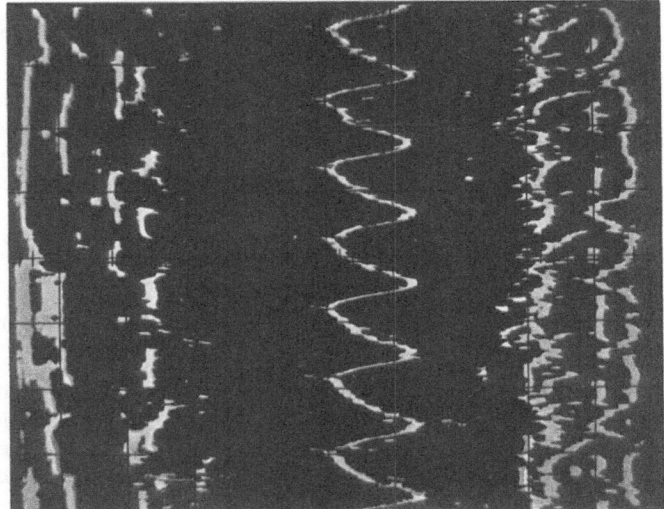

31

Anterior-Wall Placenta

Vorderwandplacenta
Placenta ventral
Localización de la placenta en cara anterior del útero
Placenta ventrale

Fig. 32. Anterior-Wall Placenta in the 39th Week of Pregnancy

Longitudinal section examination in the median line. Amnial boundary is easily recognisable by the partially broken line, as is the placenta boundary. Thickness of placenta is 4 cm. Scale divisions 1 cm. Sound frequency 2 MHz

Abb. 32. Vorderwandplacenta in der 39. Schwangerschaftswoche

Längsschnittuntersuchung in der Medianlinie. Amniale Abgrenzung durch stellenweise unterbrochene Linie sowie Placentarrand sind gut zu erkennen. Placentadicke beträgt 4 cm. Skaleneinteilung 1 cm. Schallfrequenz 2 MHZ

Fig. 32. Placenta ventral dans la 39ᵉ semaine de grossesse

Examen en coupe longitudinale dans la ligne médiane. La délimitation amniale par ligne interrompue par endroits ainsi que le bord du placenta sont bien reconnaissables. L'épaisseur du placenta est de 4 cm. Graduation 1 cm. Fréquence de son 2 MHz

Fig. 32. Placenta en cara anterior — 39 semanas de gestación

Corte longitudinal en línea media. Se puede observar el borde de la placenta y la delimitación amniótica que se representa por la línea interrumpida. El espesor de la placenta es de 4 cm. 1 división de escala = 1 cm. Frecuencia de ultrasonido = 2 MHz

Fig. 32. Placenta ventrale nella 39a settimana di gravidanza

Esame della sezione longitudinale nella linea mediana. La delimitazione amniale mediante una linea interrotta in alcuni punti, come pure il bordo della placenta sono facilmente riconoscibili. Lo spessore della placenta è di 4 cm. Graduazione 1 cm. Frequenza 2 MHZ

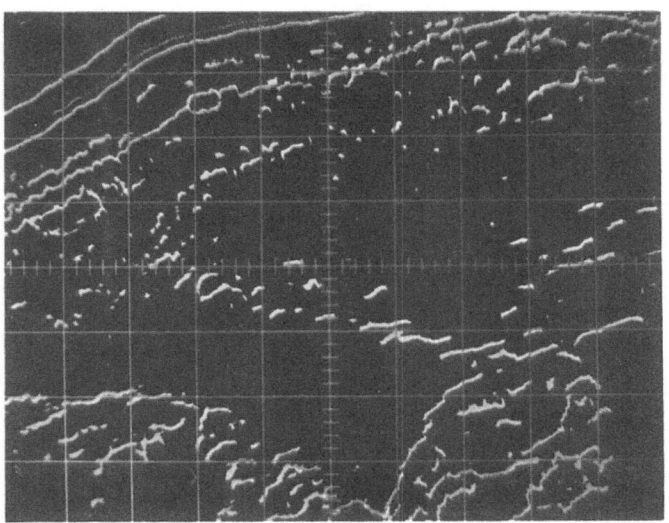

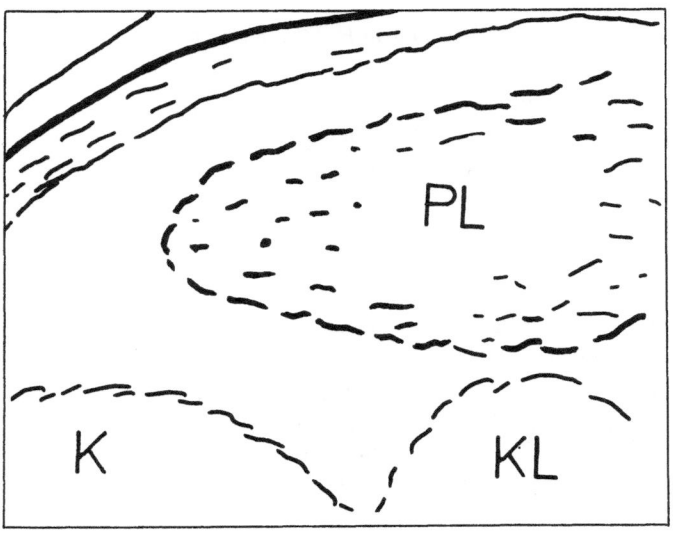

32

Fig. 33. Anterior-Wall Placenta in the 38th Week of Pregnancy

Longitudinal section to the left of the median line. Here, the full extent of the placenta can be followed. Scale divisions are 2 cm. Small members and the spinal column can be seen below the placenta

Abb. 33. Vorderwandplacenta in der 38. Schwangerschaftswoche

Längsschnitt links von der Medianlinie, hier kann man die gesamte Ausdehnung der Placenta verfolgen. Skaleneinteilung beträgt 2 cm. Unterhalb der Placenta sind kleine Teile und die Wirbelsäule sichtbar

Fig. 33. Placenta ventral dans la 38ᵉ semaine de grossesse

Coupe longitudinale à gauche de la ligne médiane; on peut suivre ici toute l'étendue du placenta. La graduation mesure 2 cm. Des parties foetales et la colonne vertébrale sont visibles en-dessous du placenta

Fig. 33. Placenta en cara anterior — 38 semanas de gestación

Corte longitudinal a la izquierda de la línea media. Se puede observar toda la extensión de la placenta y debajo de ella se encuentran las extremidades fetales y la columna vertebral. 1 división de escala = 2 cm

Fig. 33. Placenta ventrale nella 38a settimana di gravidanza

Sezione longitudinale a sinistra della linea mediana; nella figura è possibile seguire tutta l'estensione della placenta. Graduazione 2 cm. Al di sotto della placenta si intravedono estremità fetali e la colonna vertebrale

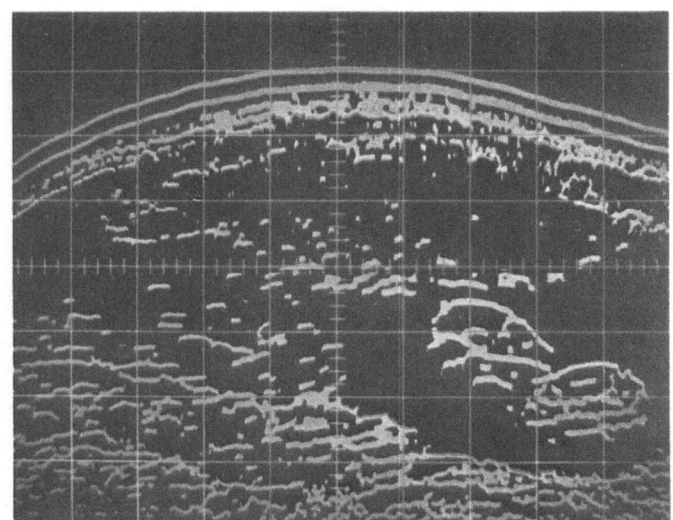

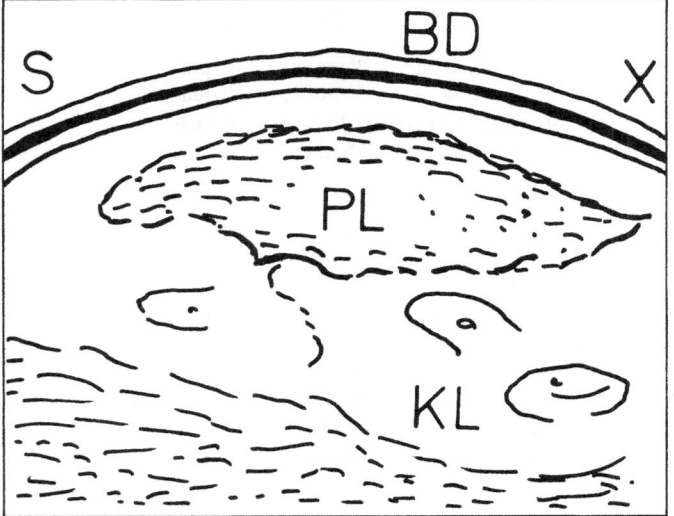

33

Fig. 34. Anterior-Wall Placenta in the 37th Week

Longitudinal section in the median line; placenta visible in full extent; scale divisions 3 cm. Small parts are visible below the placenta. Biparietal diameter is 9 cm

Abb. 34. Vorderwandplacenta in der 37. Woche

Längsschnitt in der Medianline, Placenta in gesamter Ausdehnung sichtbar, Skaleneinteilung beträgt 3 cm. Unterhalb der Placenta sind kleine Teile sichtbar. Biparietaler DM 9 cm

Fig. 34. Placenta ventral dans la 37ᵉ semaine

Coupe longitudinale dans la ligne médiane, placenta visible dans toute son étendue, la graduation mesure 3 cm. Des parties foetales sont visibles en-dessous du placenta. Diamètre bipariétal 9 cm

Fig. 34. Placenta en cara anterior — 37 semanas de gestación

Corte longitudinal en línea media. Se puede observar toda la extensión de la placenta, debajo de la cual se observan extremidades fetales. Diámetro biparietal: 9,0 cm. 1 división de escala = 3 cm

Fig. 34. Placenta ventrale nella 37a settimana

Sezione longitudinale nella linea mediana, placenta visibile in tutta la sua estensione, graduazione 3 cm. Sotto la placenta si intravedono estremità fetali. Diametro biparietale 9 cm

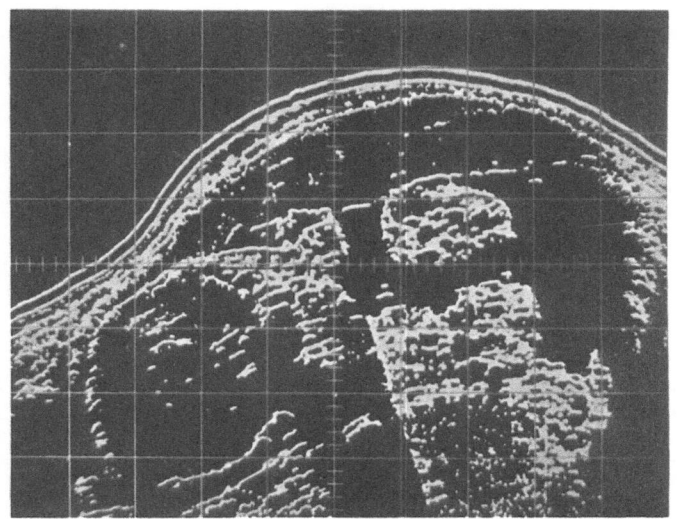

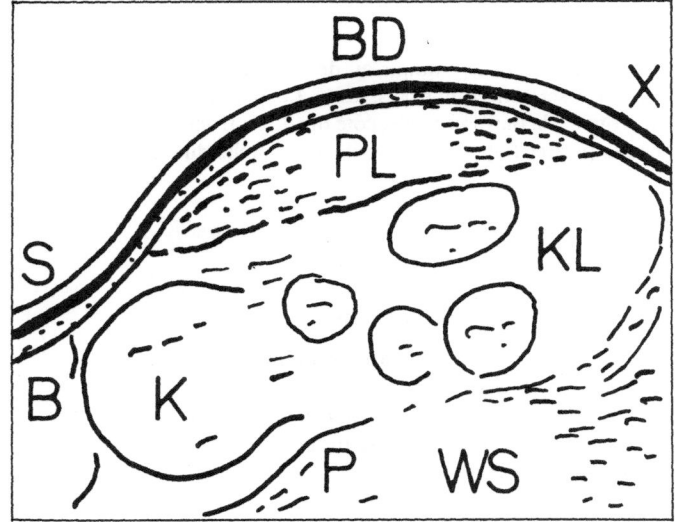

34

Fig. 35. Anterior-Wall Placenta

Cross section 2-fingers width above the navel in the 32nd week of pregnancy. Placenta is located on the right-hand side of the anterior wall. To the left of the placenta, the torso and small parts are visible

Abb. 35. Vorderwandplacenta

Querschnitt 2 QF oberhalb des Nabels bei einer Schwangerschaft in der 32. Woche. Placenta sitzt an der Vorderwand rechts seitlich. Links von der Placenta sind der Rumpf und kleine Teile sichtbar

Fig. 35. Placenta ventral

Coupe transversale 2 doigts au dessus du nombril, 32ᵉ semaine d'une grossesse. Le placenta se trouve à la paroi ventrale, côté droit. Le tronc et des parties foetales sont visibles à gauche du placenta

Fig. 35. Placenta en cara anterior

Corte transversal 2 cm. Sobre el ombligo, 32 semanas de gestación. Inserción de la placenta en el lado derecho de la cara anterior del útero. A la izquierda de la placenta se observan cuerpo y extremidades fetales

Fig. 35. Placenta ventrale

Sezione trasversale, 2 dita sopra l'ombelico, 32a settimana di gravidanza. La placenta si trova sul lato destro della parete ventrale. A sinistra della placenta si osservano il tronco e le estremità fetali

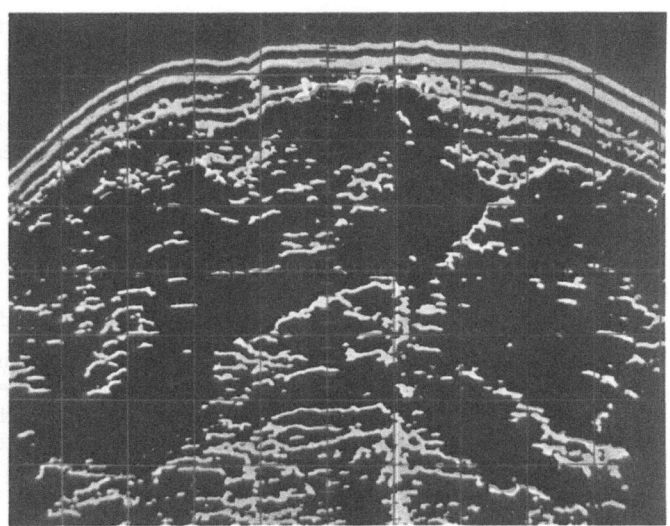

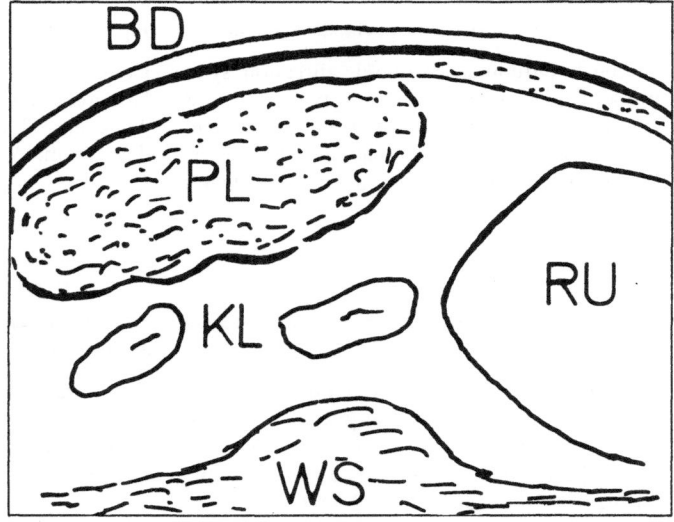

35

Fig. 36. Anterior-Wall Placenta in the 29th Week

Longitudinal section from xiphoid toward symphysis. Placenta is located on anterior wall; below placenta small parts are visible, also the bladder beyond the head. Scale divisions: 3 cm/section. Sound frequency: 2 MHz

Fig. 37. Anterior-Wall Placenta in the 29th Week

Longitudinal section in the median line of the mother, same case as Fig. 36. Scale divisions 2 cm/section. Fetal head with central echo, biparietal diameter: 7.2 cm

Abb. 36. Vorderwandplacenta in der 29. Woche

Längsschnitt, Xiphoid Richtung Symphyse, Placenta sitzt an der Vorderwand, unterhalb der Placenta sind kleine Teile sichtbar, kaudal vom Kopf die Harnblase. Skaleneinteilung pro Feld 3 cm. Schallfrequenz 2 MHZ

Abb. 37. Vorderwandplacenta in der 29. Woche

Längsschnitt in der Medianlinie der Mutter, gleicher Fall wie Abb. 36. Skaleneinteilung pro Feld 2 cm. Kindlicher Kopf mit Mittelecho, biparietaler DM 7,2 cm

Fig. 36. Placenta ventral dans la 29ᵉ semaine

Coupe longitudinale, xiphoïde direction symphyse; le placenta se trouve à la paroi ventrale. En-dessous du placenta des parties foetales sont visibles, vessie en position caudale vis-à-vis de la tête. Graduation par champ 3 cm. Fréquence de son 2 MHz

Fig. 37. Placenta ventral dans la 29ᵉ semaine

Coupe longitudinale dans la ligne médiane de la mère, même cas que l'image 36. Graduation par champ 2 cm. Tête d'enfant avec écho médian, diamètre biparétal 7,2 cm

Fig. 36. Placenta en cara anterior — 29 semanas de gestación

Corte longitudinal del xifoides en dirección pubis. Debajo de la placenta se pueden observar extremidades fetales y la vejiga materna al lado de la cabeza fetal. 1 división de escala = 3 cm. Frecuencia del ultrasonido = 2 MHz

Fig. 37. Placenta en cara anterior — 29 semanas de gestación

Mismo caso de la figura anterior. Corte longitudinal en línea media. Cabeza fetal con eco medio. Diámetro biparietal: 7,2 cm. 1 división de escala = 2 cm

Fig. 36. Placenta ventrale nella 29a settimana

Sezione longitudinale, xifoide direzione sinfisi; la placenta si trova sulla parete ventrale. Sotto la placenta si intravedono estremità fetali e la vescica in posizione caudale rispetto alla testa. Graduazione per campo 3 cm. Frequenza 2 MHZ

Fig. 37. Placenta ventrale nella 29a settimana

Sezione longitudinale nella linea mediana della madre, caso uguale a quello della fig. 36. Graduazione per campo 2 cm. Testa del bambino con eco mediano, diametro biparietale 7,2 cm

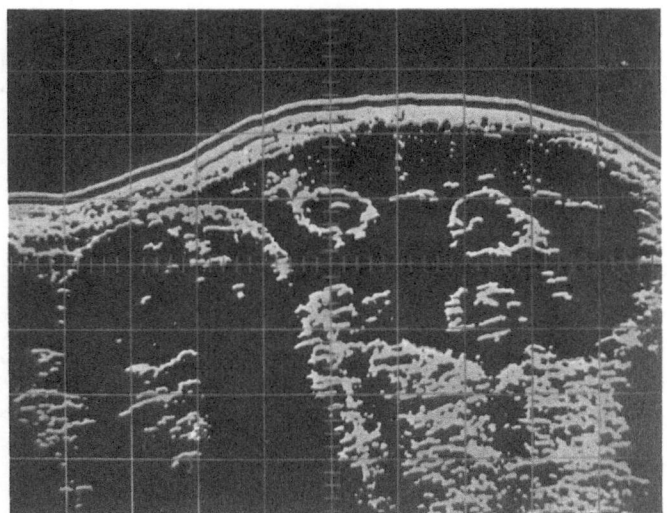

36

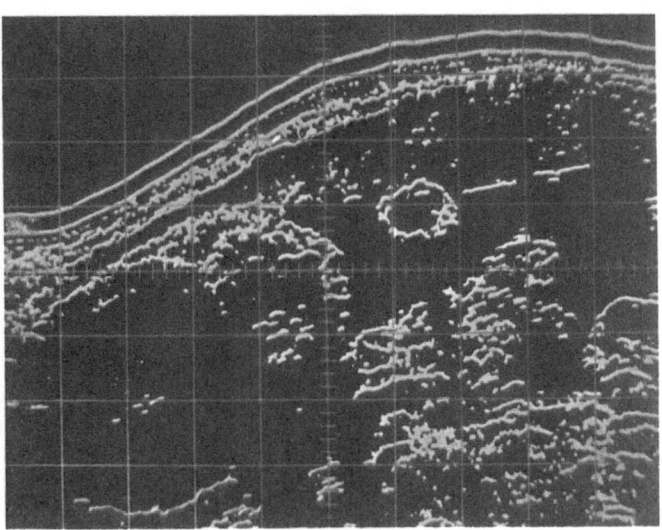

37

Fig. 38. Longitudinal Section in the Median Line

Same case as Fig. 36. Scale divisions 1 cm/section. Amnial boundary and edge of placenta can be clearly recognised; below placenta the head and other parts of child are visible

Fig. 39. Anterior-Wall Placenta in the 32nd Week

Anterior-wall placenta in cross section in the 32nd week. Placenta is on the right-hand side; torso can be seen to the left of the placenta

Abb. 38. Längsschnitt in der Medianlinie

Gleicher Fall wie Abb. 36. Skaleneinteilung pro Feld 1 cm. Amniale Begrenzung sowie Placentarrand gut zu erkennen, unterhalb der Placenta sind der Kopf und kindliche Teile sichtbar

Abb. 39. Vorderwandplacenta in der 32. Woche

Vorderwandplacenta im Querschnitt in der 32. Woche. Placenta sitzt rechts seitlich. Links von der Placenta ist der Rumpf zu erkennen

Fig. 38. Coupe longitudinale dans la ligne médiane

Même cas que l'image 36. Graduation par champ 1 cm. Délimitation amniale ainsi que le bord placentaire bien reconnaissables. La tête et des parties foetales sont visibles en-dessous du placenta

Fig. 39. Placenta ventral dans la 32ᵉ semaine

Placenta ventral en coupe transversale. Le placenta est situé latéralement à droite. A gauche du placenta on reconnaît le tronc

Fig. 38. Placenta en cara anterior

Mismo caso de la figura 36. Corte longitudinal en línea media. Se puede observar la placenta, debajo de ella la cabeza y extremidades fetales. 1 división de escala = 1 cm

Fig. 39. Placenta en cara anterior — 32 semanas de gestación

Corte transversal. La placenta se encuentra en el lado derecho. A la izquierda se observa el cuerpo fetal

Fig. 38. Sezione longitudinale nella linea mediana

Caso uguale a quello della figura 36. Graduazione per campo 1 cm. Delimitazione amniale e bordo della placenta ben riconoscibili. Sotto la placenta si intravedono la testa e le estremità fetali

Fig. 39. Placenta ventrale nella 32a settimana

Sezione trasversale della placenta ventrale nella 32a settimana. La placenta è situata sul lato destro. A sinistra della placenta si individua il tronco

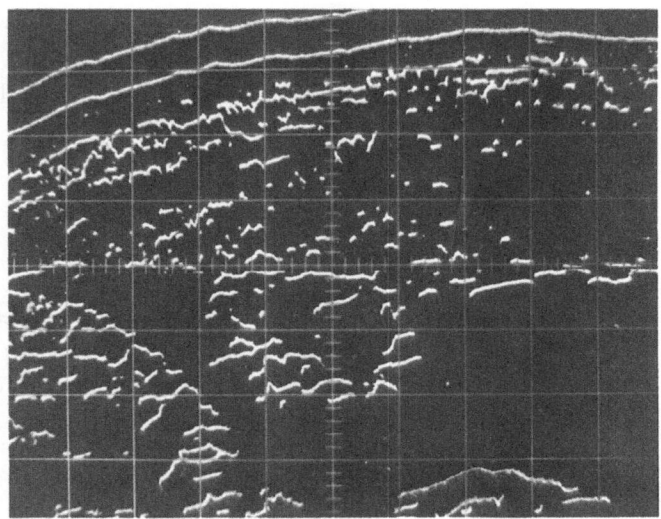

38

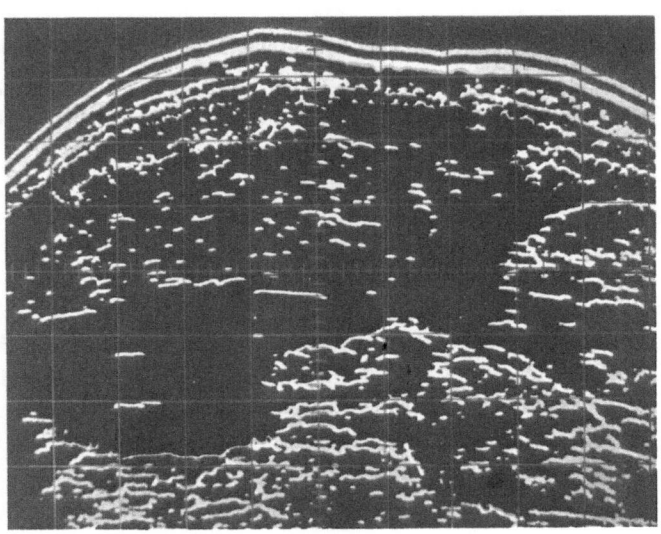

39

Fig. 40. Anterior-Wall Placenta in the 32nd Week

Longitudinal section to the right of the median line in an anterior-wall placenta. Scale divisions 2 cm/section

Fig. 41. Cross Section at Level of Navel

Same case as above. Placenta located on right; small parts clearly recognisable

Abb. 40. Vorderwandplacenta in der 32. Woche

Längsschnitt rechts von der Medianlinie bei einer Vorderwandplacenta. Skaleneinteilung pro Feld 2 cm

Abb. 41. Querschnitt in Nabelhöhe

Gleicher Fall wie oben. Placenta sitzt rechts seitlich, kleine Teile sind gut zu erkennen

Fig. 40. Placenta ventral dans la 32e semaine

Coupe longitudinale à droite de la ligne médiane d'un placenta ventral. Graduation par champ 2 cm

Fig. 41. Coupe transversale à hauteur du nombril

Le même cas que ci-dessus. Le placenta est situe latéralement à droite. Parties foetales bien distinctes

Fig. 40. Placenta en cara anterior — 32 semanas de gestación

Corte longitudinal a la derecha de la línea media. 1 división de escala = 2 cm

Fig. 41. Placenta en cara anterior

Mismo caso de la figura anterior. Corte transversal a nivel del ombligo. La placenta se encuentra en el lado derecho. Se pueden observar extremidades fetales

Fig. 40. Placenta ventrale nella 32a settimana

Sezione trasversale a destra della linea mediana in una placenta ventrale nella 32a settimana. Graduazione per campo 2 cm

Fig. 41. Sezione trasversale all'altezza dell'ombelico

Un caso uguale a quello precedente. La placenta è situata sul lato destro e si distinguono bene le estremità fetali

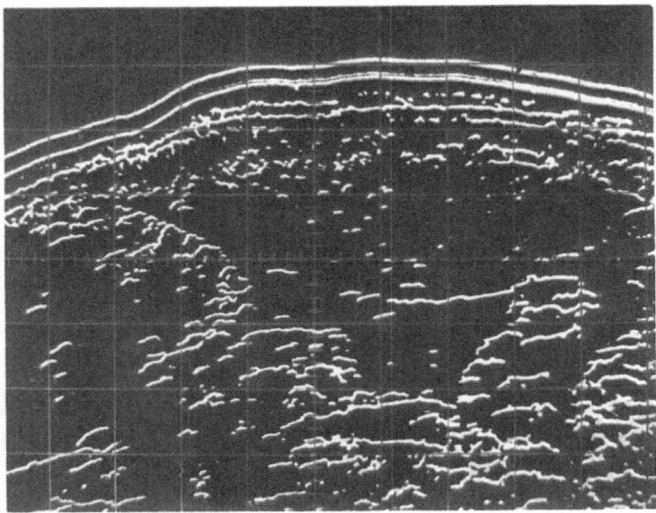

40

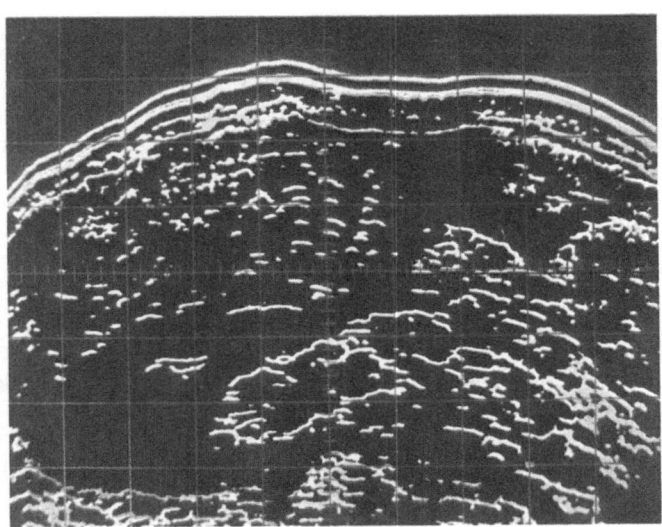

41

Fig. 42. Anterior-Wall Placenta in the 34th Week

Longitudinal section from xiphoid toward symphysis. Placenta is located on anterior wall, small parts are visible below it. Fetal head with a few dot-like echos, which can correspond to central echo and lateral reflections. Biparietal diameter is 9 cm. Scale divisions 3 cm/section

Fig. 43. Anterior-Wall Placenta in the 34th Week

Longitudinal section in the median line, same case as Fig. 42; dotted amnial boundary clearly recognisable; small parts visible below the placenta. Scale divisions: 2 cm/section

Abb. 42. Vorderwandplacenta in der 34. Woche

Längsschnitt von Xiphoid Richtung Symphyse, Placenta sitzt an der Vorderwand, darunter sind kleine Teile sichtbar, kindlicher Kopf mit einigen punktförmigen Echos, die Mittelechos und Lateralreflektionen entsprechen können, biparietaler Durchmesser beträgt 9 cm. Skaleneinteilung pro Feld 3 cm

Abb. 43. Vorderwandplacenta in der 34. Woche

Längsschnitt in der Medianlinie, gleicher Fall wie Abb. 42, strichförmige amniale Begrenzung ist gut zu erkennen, unterhalb der Placenta sind kleine Teile sichtbar. Skaleneinteilung pro Feld 2 cm

Fig. 42. Placenta ventral dans la 34e semaine

Coupe longitudinale, xiphoïde direction symphyse. Le placenta se trouve à la paroi ventrale. En-dessous, on aperçoit des parties foetales, la tête d'enfant avec quelques échos ponctuels pouvant correspondre à des échos médians ou à des réflexions latérales. Le diamètre bipariétal mesure 9 cm. Graduation par champ 3 cm

Fig. 43. Placenta ventral dans la 34e semaine

Coupe longitudinale dans la ligne médiane, même cas que l'image 42. Délimitation amniale en forme de traits bien reconnaissable. En-dessous du placenta, on aperçoit des parties foetales. Graduation par champ 2 cm

Fig. 42. Placenta en cara anterior — 34 semanas de gestación

Corte longitudinal del xifoides en dirección pubiana. La placenta se encuentra en cara anterior del útero, debajo de ella extremidades y la cabeza fetal con ecos puntiformes, los cuales pueden ser el eco medio y ecos por reflexión lateral. Diámetro biparietal: 9,0 cm. 1 división de escala = 3 cm

Fig. 43. Placenta en cara anterior

Mismo caso de la figura anterior. Corte longitudinal en línea media. Se puede observar la cavidad amniótica y la placenta, debajo de la cual se encuentran extremidades fetales. 1 división de escala = 2 cm

Fig. 42. Placenta ventrale nella 34a settimana

Sezione longitudinale, xifoide direzione sinfisi. La placenta si trova alla parete ventrale e si intravedono le estremità fetali, la testa con alcuni echi puntiformi che possono corrispondere a echi mediani o a riflessi laterali. Il diametro biparietale misura 9 cm. Graduazione per campo 3 cm

Fig. 43. Placenta ventrale nella 34a settimana

Sezione longitudinale nella linea mediana, caso uguale a quello della figura 42. La delimitazione amniale a forma di trattegio è ben riconoscibile, come pure le estremità fetali sotto la placenta. Graduazione per campo 2 cm

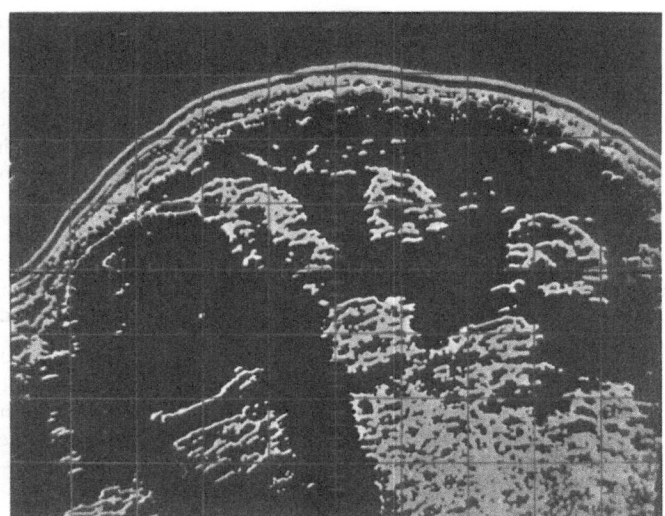

42

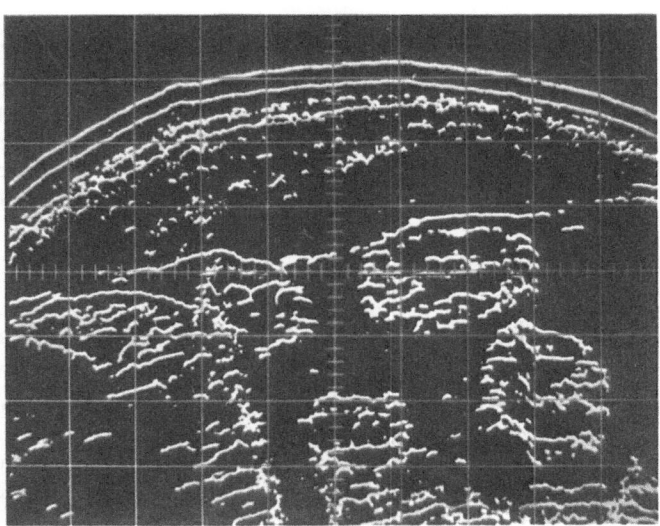

43

Fig. 44. Anterior-Wall Placenta in the 34th Week

Longitudinal section in the median line, same case as Fig. 43; Here, scale divisions 1 cm/section. Dot-like echos, which correspond to the amnial boundary. Edge of placenta is clearly recognisable. Below the placenta, part of the fetal head and small parts are visible

Fig. 45. Anterior-Wall Placenta in the 39th Week

Longitudinal section from the xiphoid toward the symphysis; placenta is located on the anterior wall. Small parts are visible below the placenta, fetal head with biparietal diameter of 9 cm. Edges of squares: 3 cm

Abb. 44. Vorderwandplacenta in der 34. Woche

Längsschnitt in der Medianlinie, gleicher Fall wie Abb. 43. Skaleneinteilung pro Feld hier 1 cm. Strichförmige Echos, die der amnialen Abgrenzung entsprechen, Placentarrand ist gut zu erkennen. Unter der Placenta sind ein Teil vom kindlichen Schädel sowie kleine Teile sichtbar

Abb. 45. Vorderwandplacenta in der 39. Woche

Längsschnittuntersuchung vom Xiphoid zur Symphyse. Placenta sitzt an der Vorderwand. Unterhalb der Placenta sind kleine Teile sichtbar, kindlicher Kopf mit biparietalem Durchmesser von 9 cm. Kantenlänge pro Feld: 3 cm

Fig. 44. Placenta ventral dans la 34ᵉ semaine

Coupe longitudinale dans la ligne médiane, même cas que l'image 43. La graduation par champ est ici de 1 cm. Echos en forme de traits correspondant à la délimitation amniale. Le bord du placenta est bien reconnaissable. En-dessous du placenta, une partie du crâne d'enfant ainsi que des parties foetales sont visibles

Fig. 45. Placenta ventral dans la 39ᵉ semaine

Examen en coupe longitudinale, du xiphoïde vers la symphyse. Le placenta se trouve à la paroi ventrale. En-dessous du placenta, on aperçoit des parties foetales. Tête d'enfant avec diamètre bipariétal de 9 cm. Longueur de côté par champ: 3 cm

Fig. 44. Placenta en cara anterior

Mismo caso de la figura 43. Corte longitudinal en línea media. Debajo de la placenta se observa parte de la cabeza fetal y extremidades fetales

Fig. 45. Placenta en cara anterior — 39 semanas de gestación

Corte longitudinal del xifoides al pubis. Debajo de la placenta se pueden observar cabeza y extremidades fetales. Diámetro biparietal: 9,0 cm. 1 división de escala = 3 cm

Fig. 44. Placenta ventrale nella 34a settimana

Sezione longitudinale nella linea mediana, caso uguale a quello della figura 43. Graduazione per campo 1 cm. Eco a forma di tratteggio che corrispondono alla delimitazione amniale. Il bordo della placenta è ben riconoscibile e al di sotto di essa si osservano una parte del cranio e estremità fetali

Fig. 45. Placenta ventrale nella 39a settimana

Esama in sezione longitudinale dallo xifoide verso la sinfisi. La Placenta si trova sulla parete ventrale. Sotto la placenta si osservano estremità fetali. La testa ha un diametro biparietale di 9 cm. Lunghezza del lato per campo 3 cm

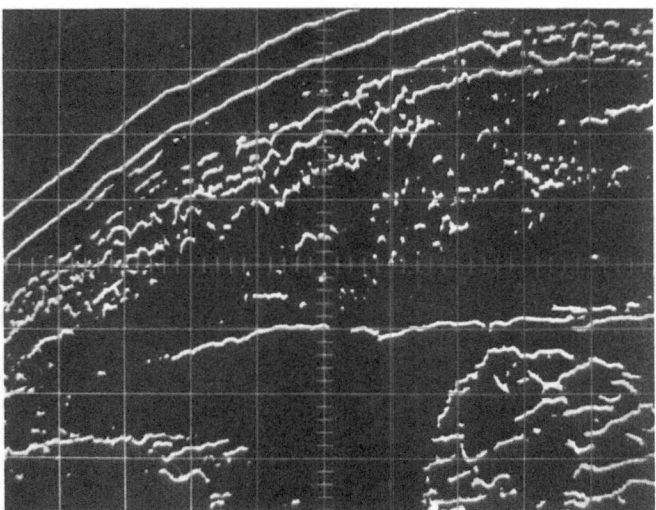

44

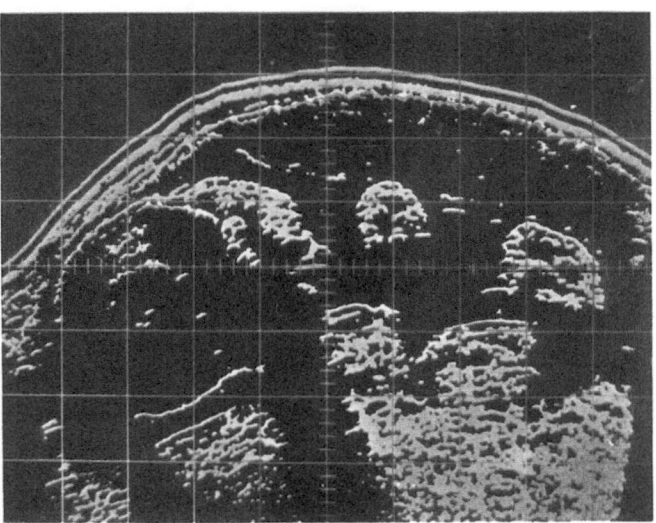

45

Fig. 46. Anterior-Wall Placenta in the 39th Week

Longitudinal section in the median line, same case as Fig. 45; In the center of the placenta, toward the posterior wall, small dotted echos can be seen, which could correspond to the umbilical cord. Scale divisions: 2 cm

Fig. 47. Anterior-Wall Placenta in the 39th Week

Same case as Fig. 46; scale divisions are 1 cm/section; amnial boundary and edge of placenta are very well defined; cotyledons can be seen between the fetus and the maternal part of the placenta

Abb. 46. Vorderwandplacenta in der 39. Woche

Längsschnitt in der Medianlinie, gleicher Fall wie Abb. 45, in der Mitte der Placenta Richtung Hinterwand sieht man kleine strichförmige Echos, die der Nabelschnur entsprechen könnten. Skaleneinteilung 2 cm

Abb. 47. Vorderwandplacenta in der 39. Woche

Gleicher Fall wie Abb. 46, Skaleneinteilung beträgt pro Feld 1 cm, amniale Abgrenzung sowie Placentarrand sind hier sehr gut abzugrenzen, zwischen kindlichem und mütterlichem Teil der Placenta sind Cotyledonen zu erkennen

Fig. 46. Placenta ventral dans la 39ᵉ semaine

Coupe longitudinale dans la ligne médiane, même cas que l'image 45. Au milieu du placenta, direction paroi dorsale, on aperçoit des petits échos en forme de traits qui peuvent correspondre au cordon ombilical. Graduation 2 cm

Fig. 47. Placenta ventral dans la 39ᵉ semaine

Même cas que l'image 46. La graduation par champ mesure 1 cm. La délimitation amniale ainsi que le bord placentaire se distinguent ici très nettement. On aperçoit des cotylédons entre la partie enfant et la partie mère du placenta

Fig. 46. Placenta en cara anterior.

Mismo caso de la figura 45. Corte longitudinal. En el centro de la placenta, hacia la cara posterior del útero se observan pequeños ecos lineares que pueden corresponder al cordón umbilical. 1 división de escala = 2 cm

Fig. 47. Placenta en cara anterior

Mismo caso de la figura 46. Entre la parte materna y la parte fetal de la placenta se pueden observar ecos que corresponden a cotiledones. 1 división de escala = 1 cm

Fig. 46. Placenta ventrale nella 39a settimana

Sezione longitudinale nella linea mediana, caso uguale a quello della figura 45. Nel mezzo della placenta in direzione della parete dorsale si osservano piccoli echi a tratteggio che potrebbero corrispondere al cordone ombelicale. Graduazione 2 cm

Fig. 47. Placenta ventrale nella 39a settimana

Caso uguale a quello della figura 46, graduazione per campo di 1 cm. La delimitazione amniale e il bordo della placenta sono ben riconoscibili. Fra la parte del bambino e la parte della madre della placenta si osservano dei cotiledoni

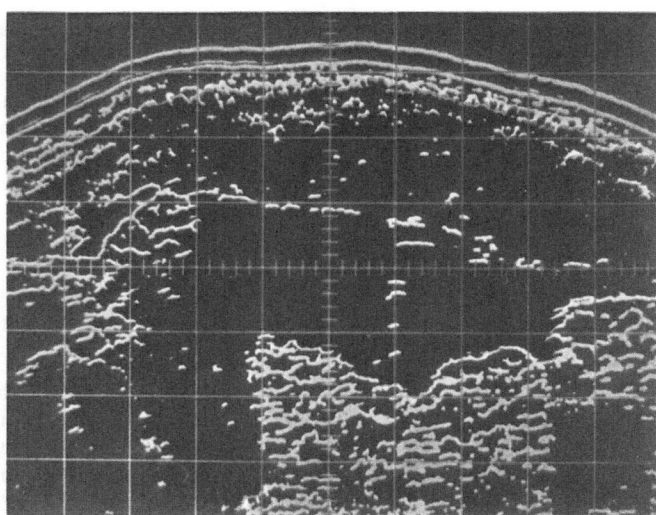

46

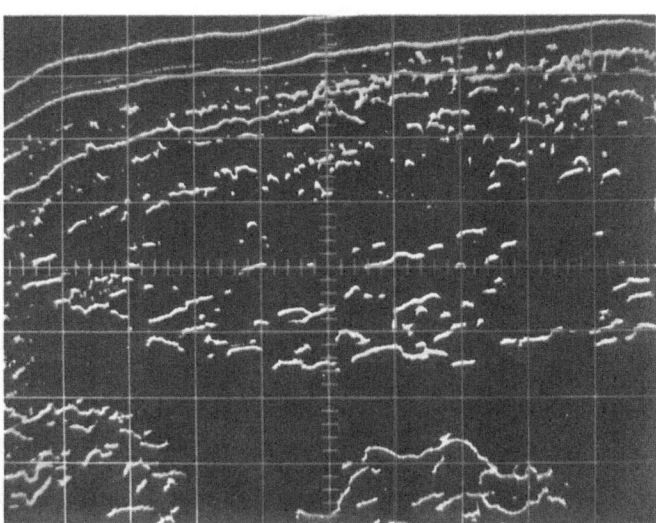

47

Posterior-Wall Placenta

Hinterwandplacenta
Placenta dorsal
Localización de la placenta en cara posterior del útero
Placenta dorsale

Fig. 48. Posterior-Wall Placenta in the 30th Week

Longitudinal section to the left of the median line; between the fetus' and the mother's side of the placenta are multiple dots and dotted echos, and cotyledons are also recognisable. Length of sides of squares: 2 cm. Sound frequency: 2 MHz

Abb. 48. Hinterwandplacenta in der 30. Woche

Längsschnitt links von der Medianlinie, zwischen kindlicher und mütterlicher Seite der Placenta befinden sich multiple Punkte und strichförmige Echos, ebenfalls sind Cotyledonen zu erkennen. Kantenlänge pro Feld 2 cm. Schallfrequenz 2 MHZ

Fig. 48. Placenta dorsal dans la 30ᵉ semaine

Coupe longitudinale à gauche de la ligne médiane. Entre le côté enfant et le côté mère du placenta se trouvent des multiples points et échos en forme de traits. On aperçoit également des cotylédons. Longueur de côté par champ 2 cm. Fréquence de son 2 MHz

Fig. 48. Placenta en cara posterior. Embarazo de 30 semanas

Corte longitudinal a la izquierda de la línea media. Entre la parte materna y la parte fetal de la placenta se pueden observar ecos que corresponden a cotiledones. 1 división de escala = 2 cm. Frecuencia del ultrasonido = 2 MHz

Fig. 48. Placenta dorsale nella 30a settimana

Sezione longitudinale a sinistra della linea mediana. Fra il lato bambino e il lato madre della placenta si sono molti punti e echi a forma di tratteggio e si intravedono dei cotiledoni. Lunghezza del lato per campo 2 cm. Frequenza 2 MHZ

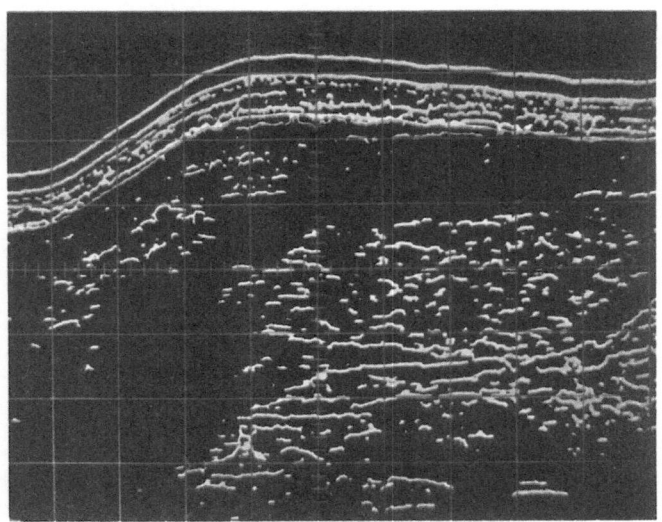

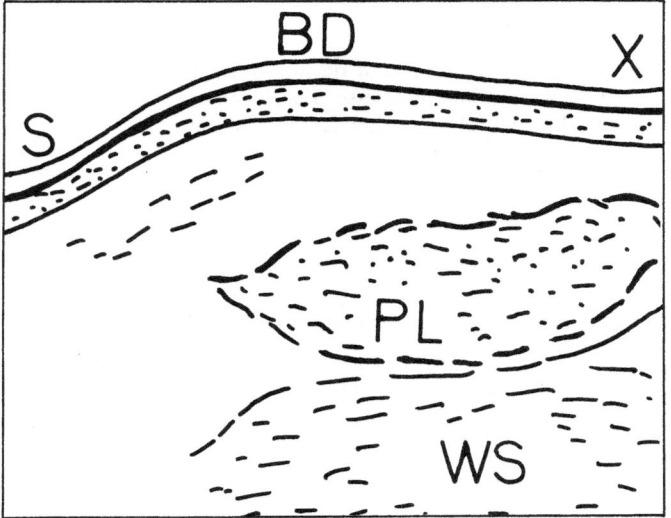

48

Fig. 49. Posterior-Wall Placenta

Cross section at the level of the navel in 30th week of pregnancy. Placenta easily recognisable on the posterior wall. Scale divisions: 2 cm/section

Abb. 49. Hinterwandplacenta

Querschnitt in Nabelhöhe bei einer Gravidität in der 30. Woche. Placenta an der Hinterwand gut zu erkennen. Skaleneinteilung pro Feld 2 cm

Fig. 49. Placenta dorsal

Coupe transversale à hauteur du nombril dans la 30ᵉ semaine d'une grossesse. Le placenta à la paroi dorsale est bien reconnaissable. Graduation par champ 2 cm

Fig. 49. Placenta en cara posterior. Embarazo de 30 semanas

Corte transversal a nivel de ombligo. 1 división de escala = 2 cm

Fig. 49. Placenta dorsale

Sezione all'altezza dell'ombelico nella 30a settimana di gravidanza. La placenta è ben riconoscibile sulla parete dorsale. Graduazione per campo 2 cm

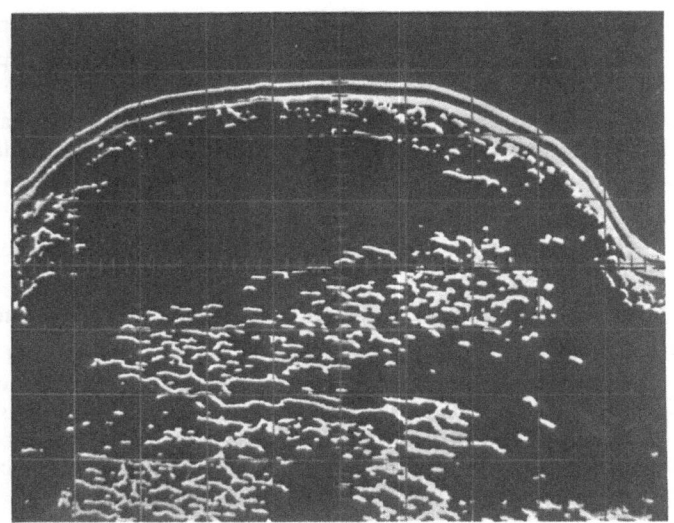

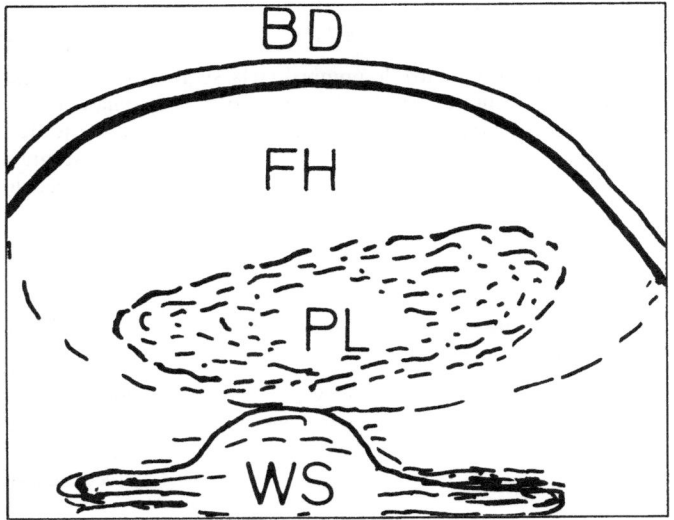

49

Fig. 50. Posterior-Wall Placenta in the 24th Week

Cross section between navel and symphysis in a 24-week pregnancy. Placenta is located on the posterior wall; cranium and torso can be seen above the placenta

Fig. 51. Posterior-Wall Placenta in the 24th Week

Same case as Fig. 50, but in longitudinal section to the left of the median line. The full extent of the placenta can be traced. Placenta is $4^{1}/_{2}$ cm thick. Scale divisions: 2 cm. Sound frequency: 2 MHz

Abb. 50. Hinterwandplacenta in der 24. Woche

Querschnitt zwischen Nabel und Symphyse bei einer 24wöchigen Gravidität. Placenta sitzt an der Hinterwand. Oberhalb der Placenta sind Schädel und Rumpf zu erkennen

Abb. 51. Hinterwandplacenta in der 24. Woche

Gleicher Fall wie Abb. 50, jedoch im Längsschnitt links von der Medianlinie. Placenta ist in ganzer Ausdehnung zu verfolgen, Placentadicke beträgt $4^{1}/_{2}$ cm, Skaleneinteilung 2 cm. Schallfrequenz 2 MHZ

Fig. 50. Placenta dorsal dans la 24ᵉ semaine

Coupe transversale entre le nombril et la symphyse. Le placenta est situé à la paroi dorsale. On aperçoit le crâne et le tronc audessus du placenta

Fig. 51. Placenta dorsal dans la 24ᵉ semaine

Même cas que l'image 50, mais en coupe longitudinale à gauche de la ligne médiane. On peut suivre toute l'étendue du placenta. L'épaisseur du placenta est de 4-$^{1}/_{2}$ cm. Graduation 2 cm. Fréquence de son 2 MHz

Fig. 50. Placenta en cara posterior — Embarazo de 24 semanas

Corte transversal entre xifoides y pubis. Sobre la placenta se observa la cabeza y el cuerpo fetal

Fig. 51. Placenta en cara posterior

Mismo caso de la figura anterior. Corte longitudinal a la izquierda de la línea media. La placenta se puede observar en toda su extensión, su espesor es de 4,5 cm. 1 división de escala = 2 cm. Frecuencia del ultrasonido = 2 MHz

Fig. 50. Placenta dorsale nella 24a settimana

Sezione trasversale fra l'ombelico e la sinfisi. Gravidanza di 24 settimane. La placenta è situata sulla parete dorsale. Si osserva sopra la placenta il cranio e il tronco

Fig. 51. Placenta dorsale nella 24a settimana

Caso uguale a quello della fig. 50, ma in sezione longitudinale a sinistra della linea mediana. E' possibile seguire tutta l'estensione della placenta, il cui spessore è di $4^{1}/_{2}$ cm. Graduazione 2 cm. Frequenza 2 MHZ

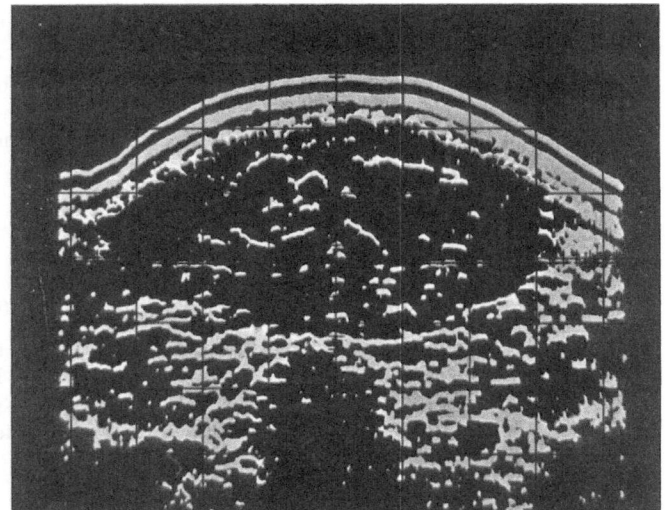

50

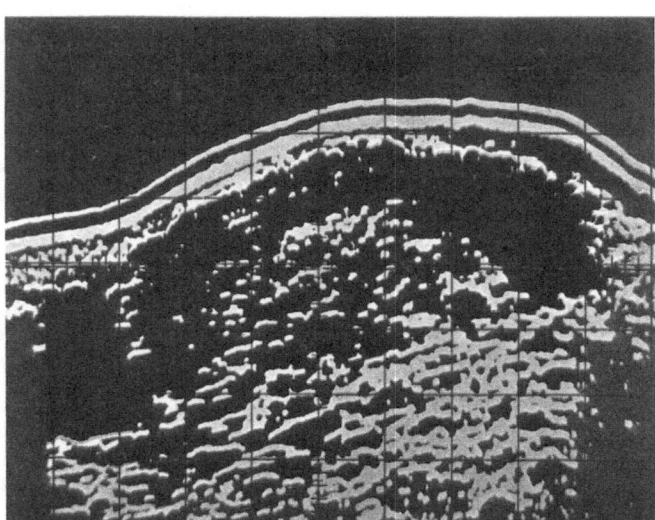

51

Fig. 52. Posterior-Wall Placenta in the 37th Week

Cross section 1-finger width below navel; placenta located on posterior wall to the left with very sharp amnial boundary. Parts of the fetus can be seen to the right of the placenta. Scale divisions: 2 cm

Fig. 53. Posterior-Wall Placenta in the 34th Week

Longitudinal section to the right of the median line. Size of squares: 3 cm. Placenta on the posterior wall; uterus well definable. Bladder is visible beyond the uterus. Sound frequency: 2 MHz

Abb. 52. Hinterwandplacenta in der 37. Woche

Querschnitt 1 QF unterhalb des Nabels. Placenta sitzt an der Hinterwand links mit sehr scharfer amnialer Abgrenzung. Rechts von der Placenta sind fetale Teile erkennbar. Skaleneinteilung 2 cm

Abb. 53. Hinterwandplacenta in der 34. Woche

Längsschnitt rechts von der Medianlinie. Kantenlänger pro Feld 3 cm. Placenta an der Hinterwand, Uterus gut abgrenzbar. Caudal vom Uterus ist die Harnblase sichtbar. Schallfrequenz 2 MHZ

Fig. 52. Placenta dorsal dans la 37ᵉ semaine

Coupe transversale 1 doigt en-dessous du nombril. Le placenta se trouve au côté gauche de la paroi dorsale avec une délimitation amniale très marquée. A droite du placenta on aperçoit des parties foetales. Graduation 2 cm

Fig. 53. Placenta dorsal dans la 34ᵉ semaine

Coupe longitudinale à droite de la ligne médiane. Longueur de côté par champ 3 cm. Placenta à la paroi dorsale. Utérus bien délimité. La vessie est visible en direction caudale de l'utérus. Fréquence de son 2 MHz

Fig. 52. Placenta en cara posterior — Embarazo de 37 semanas

Corte transversal a 1 cm debajo del ombligo. La placenta se encuentra inserta en el lado posterior izquierdo de la matriz. A la derecho se pueden observar extremidades fetales. 1 división de escala = 2 cm

Fig. 53. Placenta en cara posterior — Embarazo de 34 semanas

Corte longitudinal a la derecha de la línea media. Debajo del útero se encuentra la vejiga. 1 división de escala = 3 cm. Frecuencia del ultrasonido = 2 MHz

Fig. 52. Placenta dorsale nella 37a settimana

Sezione trasversale un dito sotto l'ombelico. La placenta si trova sul lato sinistro della parete dorsale con una delimitazione amniale molto netta, a destra della placenta si individuano estremità fetali. Graduazione 2 cm

Fig. 53. Placenta dorsale nella 34a settimana

Sezione longitudinale a destra della linea mediana. Lunghezza del lato per camp 3 cm. Placenta situata alla parete dorsale, utero ben delimitato. La vescica è visibile in direzione caudale rispetto all'utero. Frequenza 2 MHZ

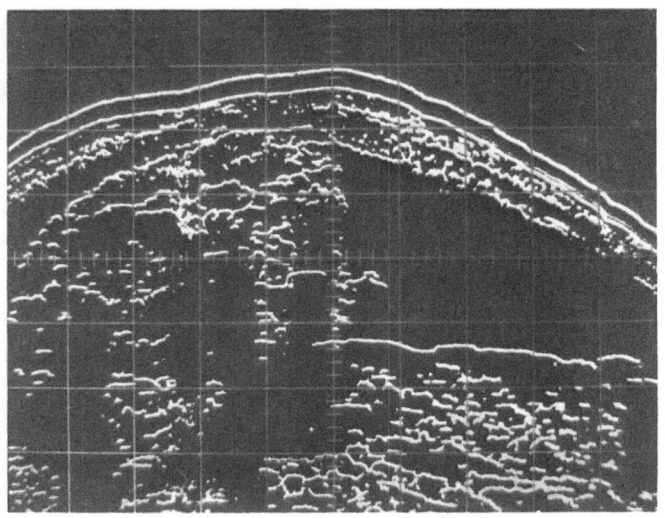

52

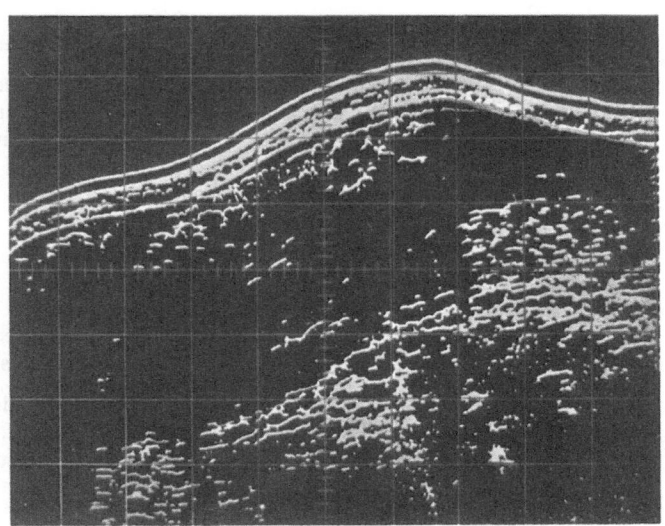

53

Fig. 54. Posterior-Wall Placenta in the 34th Week

Cross section 2-fingers' width above the navel, same case as Fig. 53. Placenta located on the posterior wall to the right; beside the placenta is the child's head in breech presentation. Central echo is clearly visible; biparietal diameter is 8 cm. Size of squares 2 cm

Fig. 55. Posterior-Wall Placenta in the 34th Week

Same case as Fig. 54; here the sides of the sections are 2 cm long. Extent and thickness of placenta can be measured with no difficulty

Abb. 54. Hinterwandplacenta in der 34. Woche

Querschnitt 2 Querfinger oberhalb des Nabels, gleicher Fall wie Abb. 53. Placenta sitzt an der Hinterwand rechts, neben Placenta liegt kindlicher Kopf bei Beckenendlage. Mittelecho ist deutlich sichtbar, biparietaler DM beträgt 8 cm, Kantenlänge pro Feld 2 cm

Abb. 55. Hinterwandplacenta in der 34. Woche

Gleicher Fall wie Abb. 54, hier beträgt die Kantenlänge pro Feld 2 cm, Placentaausdehnung und -dicke können ohne Mühe gemessen werden

Fig. 54. Placenta dorsal dans la 34ᵉ semaine

Coupe transversale 2 doigts au-dessus du nombril, même cas que l'image 53. Le placenta se trouve au côté droit de la paroi dorsale. A côté du placenta se trouve la tête de l'enfant, en présentation du siège. L'écho médian est nettement visible. Le diamètre bipariétal est de 8 cm. Longueur de côté par champ 2 cm

Fig. 55. Placenta dorsal dans la 34ᵉ semaine

Même cas que l'image 54. La longueur de côté par champ est ici de 2 cm. L'étendue et l'épaisseur placentaires peuvent être mesurées sans difficultés

Fig. 54. Placenta en cara posterior — Embarazo de 34 semanas

Mismo caso de la figura 53. Corte transversal a 2 cm. sobre el ombligo. La placenta se encuentra inserta en el lado posterior derecho. Lateralmente se encuentra la cabeza fetal con el eco medio. Diámetro biparietal: 8,0 cm. 1 división de escala = 2 cm

Fig. 55. Placenta en cara posterior — Embarazo de 34 semanas

Mismo caso de la figura 54. El tamaño y espesor de la placenta puede medirse sin dificultad. 1 división de escala = 2 cm

Fig. 54. Placenta dorsale nella 34a settimana

Sezione trasversale 2 dita sopra l'ombelico, caso uguale a quello della figura 53. La placenta si trova sul lato destro della parete dorsale. Accanto alla placenta la testa del bambino con presentazione pelvica. L'eco mediano è ben visibile, il diametro biparietale è di 8 cm. Lunghezza del lato per campo 2 cm

Fig. 55. Placenta dorsale nella 34a settimana

Caso uguale a quello della figura 54. La lunghezza del lato per campo è in questo caso di 2 cm. L'estensione e lo spessore della placenta possono essere misurati senza difficoltà

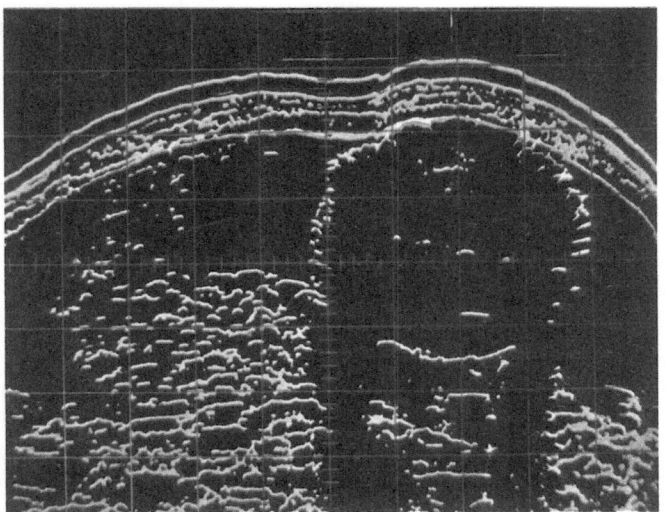

54

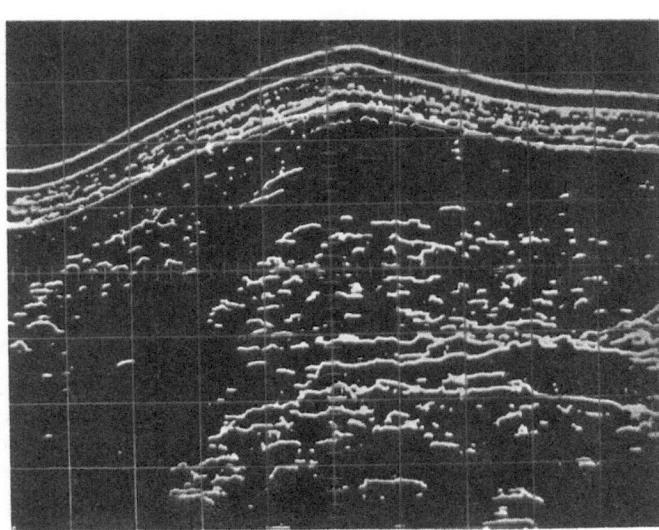

55

Fundal Placenta

Fundusplacenta
Placenta du fond utérin
Localización de la placenta en el fondo uterino
Placenta del fondo uterino

Fig. 56. Fundal Placenta

Longitudinal section in the median line in the 28th week of pregnancy. Placenta is located on the anterior wall, fundus, and posterior wall

Abb. 56. Fundusplacenta

Längsschnitt in der Medianlinie bei einer Schwangerschaft in der 28. Woche. Placenta sitzt an Vorderwand, Fundus und Hinterwand

Fig. 56. Placenta du fond utérin

Coupe longitudinale dans la ligne médiane dans la 28ᵉ semaine d'une grossesse. Le placenta se trouve à la paroi ventrale, au fond et à la paroi dorsale

Fig. 56. Placenta en fondo uterino

Corte longitudinal en línea media. Embarazo de 28 semanas. Inserción de la placenta en cara anterior, fondo y cara posterior del útero

Fig. 56. Placenta del fondo uterino

Sezione longitudinale nella linea mediana alla 28a settimana di gravidanza. La placenta si trova sulla parete ventrale sul fondo e sulla parte dorsale

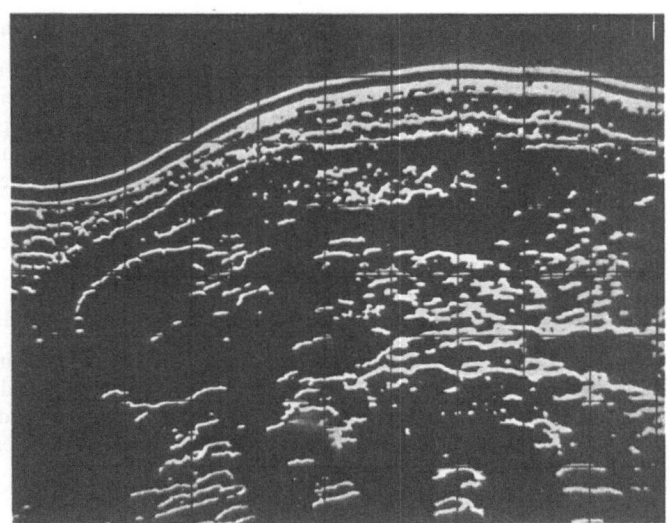

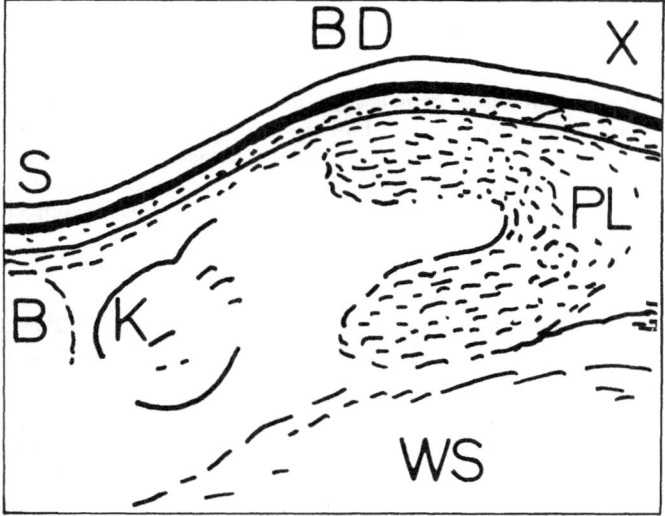

56

Fig. 57. Fundal Placenta in the 30 Week

Longitudinal section in the median line in the 30th week of pregnancy. Placenta is located at the fundus, fetal parts can be seen below the placenta. Scale divisions: 2 cm/section

Fig. 58. Fundal Placenta in the 29th Week

Longitudinal section in the median line of the mother. Placenta is located on the anterior wall, fundus, and posterior wall. The fetal cranium can be seen in front of the placenta. Scale divisions: 3 cm per section

Abb. 57. Fundusplacenta in der 30. Woche

Längsschnitt in der Medianlinie bei einer Schwangerschaft in der 30. Woche. Placenta sitzt am Fundus, unterhalb der Placenta sind fetale Teile erkennbar. Skaleneinteilung pro Feld 2 cm

Abb. 58. Fundusplacenta in der 29. Woche

Längsschnitt in der Medianlinie der Mutter. Placenta sitzt an der Vorderwand, Fundus und Hinterwand. Vor der Placenta ist der kindliche Schädel zu erkennen. Skaleneinteilung pro Feld 3 cm

Fig. 57. Placenta du fond utérin dans la 30ᵉ semaine

Coupe longitudinale dans la ligne médiane. Le placenta se trouve au fond. En-dessous du placenta on reconnaît des parties foetales. Graduation par champ 2 cm

Fig. 58. Placenta du fond utérin dans la 29ᵉ semaine

Coupe longitudinale dans la ligne médiane de la mère. Le placenta se trouve à la paroi ventrale, au fond et à la paroi dorsale. On aperçoit le crâne d'enfant devant le placenta. Graduation par champ 3 cm

Fig. 57. Placenta en fondo uterino — Embarazo de 30 semanas

Corte longitudinal en linea media. Debajo de la placenta se encuentran extremidades fetales. 1 división de escala = 2 cm

Fig. 58. Placenta en fondo uterino — Embarazo de 29 semanas

Corte longitudinal en línea media. Inserción de la placenta en cara anterior, fondo y cara posterior de la matriz. Delante de la placenta se encuentra la cabeza fetal. 1 división de escala = 3 cm

Fig. 57. Placenta del fondo uterino nella 30a settimana

Sezione longitudinale nella linea mediana alla 30a settimana di gravidanza. La placenta si trova sul fondo e sotto di essa sono riconoscibili parti fetali. Graduazione per campo 2 cm

Fig. 58. Placenta del fondo uterino nella 29a settimana

Sezione longitudinale nella linea mediana della madre. La placenta si trova sulla parete ventrale, sul fondo e sulla parete dorsale. Davanti alla placenta si osserva il cranio. Graduazione per campo 3 cm

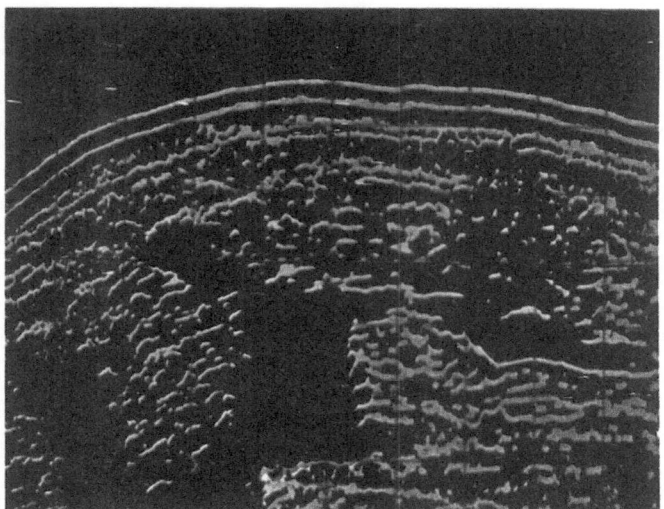

57

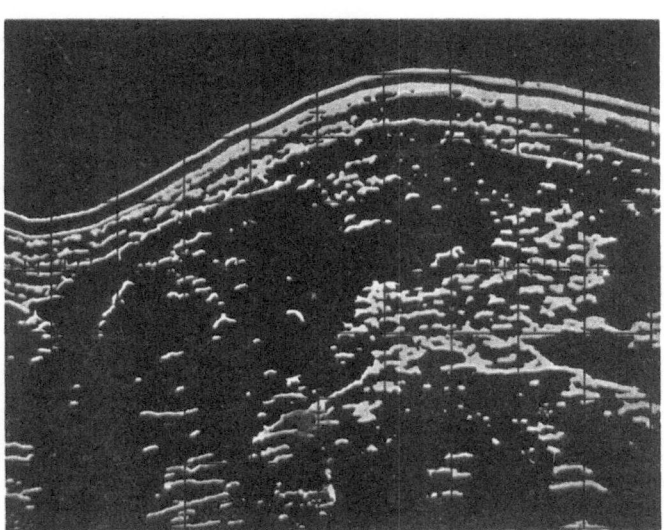

58

Fig. 59. Cross section with a Fundal Placenta in the 29th Week

Same case as Fig. 58; Placenta can be seen partly on the anterior and partly on the posterior wall

Abb. 59. Querschnitt bei einer Fundusplacenta in der 29. Woche

Gleicher Fall wie Abb. 58. Placenta z.T. an Vorder-, z.T. an Hinterwand zu erkennen

Fig. 59. Coupe transversale d'un placenta du fond utérin dans la 29ᵉ semaine

Même cas que l'image 58. On distingue le placenta en partie à la paroi ventrale et en partie à la paroi dorsale

Fig. 59. Placenta en fondo uterino

Mismo caso de la figura 58. Corte transversal. Se puede reconocer parcialmente la placenta en cara anterior y posterior del útero

Fig. 59. Sezione trasversale di una placenta del fondo uterino nella 29a settimana

Caso uguale a quello della fig. 58. Si osserva la placenta in parte sulla parete ventrale e in parte sulla parete dorsale

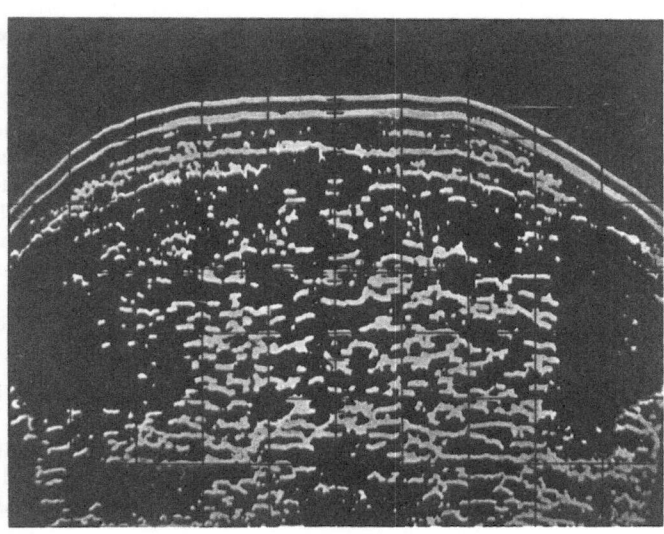

59

Placenta Praevia

Placenta praevia
Placenta praevia
Placenta previa
Placenta previa

Fig. 60. Placenta Praevia Totalis with Breech Presentation

Longitudinal section in the median line in the case of a placenta praevia totalis in the 30th week. The placenta is located on the posterior wall of the uterus and completely overlaps the cervical canal. It even reaches to the anterior wall. Scale divisions are 3 cm/section

Abb. 60. Placenta praevia totalis bei Beckenendlage

Längsschnitt in der Medianlinie bei einer Placenta praevia totalis in der 30. Woche. Placenta sitzt an der Uterushinterwand und überlappt den Cervicalkanal völlig. Sie reicht sogar bis zur Vorderwand. Skaleneinteilung pro Feld 3 cm

Fig. 60. Placenta praevia totalis avec présentation par le siège

Coupe longitudinale dans la ligne médiane. Placenta praevia totalis dans la 30e semaine. Le placenta se trouve à la paroi dorsale de l'utérus et recouvre entièrement la cavité du col utérin. Il s'étend même à la paroi ventrale. Graduation par champ 3 cm

Fig. 60. Placenta previa total y presentación podálica — Embarazo de 30 semanas

Corte longitudinal en línea media. Inserción de la placenta en cara posterior, sobre el orificio interno y cara anterior del útero. 1 división de escala = 3 cm

Fig. 60. Placenta previa totale in caso di posizione podalica

Sezione longitudinale sulla linea mediana in caso di Placenta previa totale nella 30a settimana. La placenta si trova sulla parete posteriore dell'utero e ostruisce completamente il canale cervicale, arrivando a toccare persino la parete anteriore. Graduazione della scala: 3 cm per campo

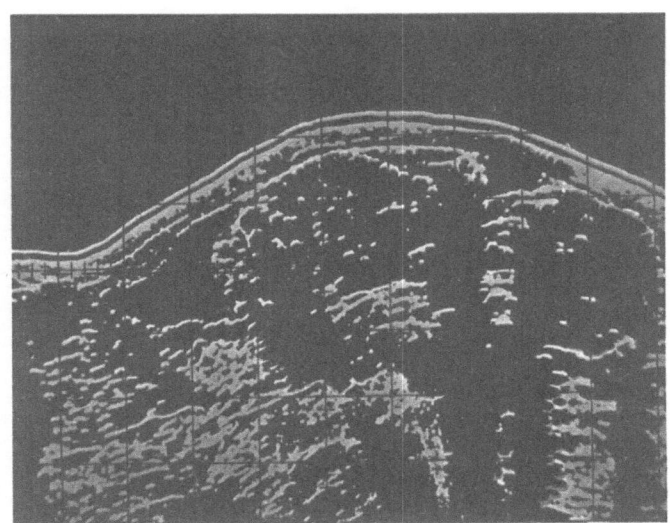

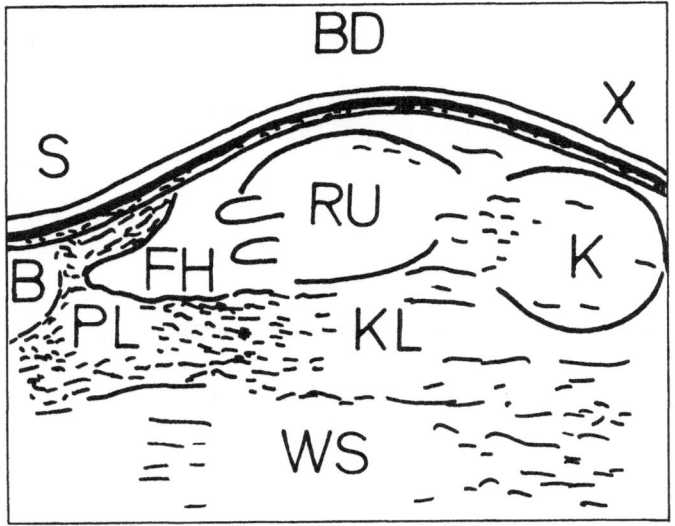

60

Fig. 61. Placenta Praevia Totalis with Breech Presentation

Same case as Fig. 60, but with scale 1 cm/section. The internal orifice is covered by the placenta. Sound frequency: 2 MHz

Abb. 61. Placenta praevia totalis bei Beckenendlage

Gleicher Fall wie Abb. 60, jedoch mit Kantenlänge 1 cm pro Feld. Der innere Muttermund ist von der Placenta bedeckt. Schallfrequenz 2 MHZ

Fig. 61. Placenta praevia totalis avec présentation par le siège

Même cas que l'image 60, mais avec longueur de côté de 1 cm par champ. L'orifice interne de l'utérus est recouvert par le placenta. Fréquence de son 2 MHz

Fig. 61. Placenta previa total y presentación podálica

Mismo caso de la figura 60, pero con 1 división de escala = 2 cm. El orificio interno es recubierto totalemente por la placenta. Frecuencia del ultrasonido = 2 MHz

Fig. 61. Placenta previa totale in caso di presentazione podalica

Caso uguale a quello della Fig. 60. Lunghezza del lato: 1 cm. per campo. Bocca uterina interna quasi del tutto coperta dalla placenta. Frequenza 2 MHZ

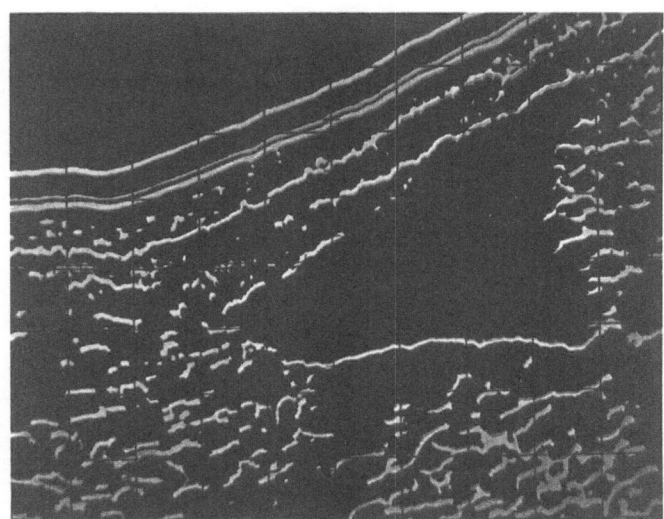

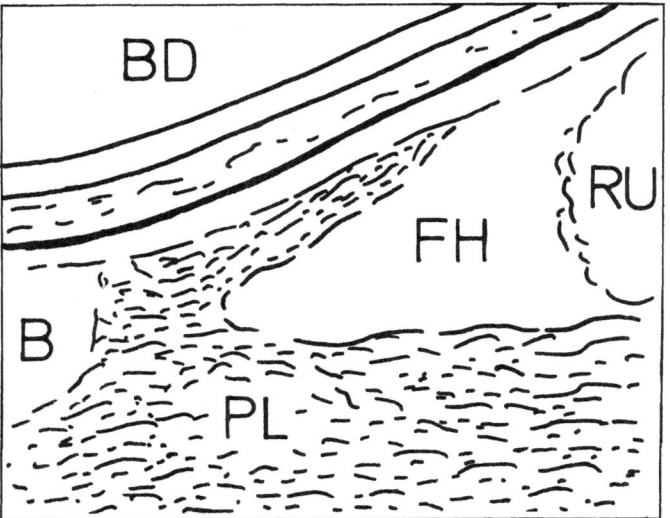

Fig. 62. Placenta Praevia Totalis

Longitudinal section in the median line with a placenta praevia totalis in the 36th week. The placenta is inserted on the anterior wall of the uterus and completely overlaps the cervical-canal. It extends as far as the posterior wall. The bladder is located below. Scale divisions are 2 cm/section

Abb. 62. Placenta praevia totalis

Längsschnitt in der Medianlinie bei einer Placenta praevia totalis in der 36. Woche. Die Placenta inseriert an der Uterusvorderwand und überlappt den Cervicalkanal völlig. Sie reicht bis zur Uterushinterwand. Caudal liegt die Harnblase. Skaleneinteilung pro Feld 2 cm

Fig. 62. Placenta praevia totalis

Coupe longitudinale dans la ligne médiane. Placenta praevia totalis dans la 36ᵉ semaine. Le placenta s'insère sur la paroi ventrale de l'utérus et recouvre entièrement la cavité du col utérin. Il s'étend jusqu'à la paroi dorsale de l'utérus. Vessie en direction caudale. Graduation par champ 2 cm

Fig. 62. Placenta previa total

Corte longitudinal en línea media. Embarazo de 36 semanas. La placenta está inserta en cara anterior del útero, cubre totalmente el orificio interno y continua en cara posterior. 1 división de escala = 2 cm

Fig. 62. Placenta previa totale

Sezione longitudinale sulla linea mediana in caso di placenta previa totale nella 36a settimana. La placenta, partendo dalla parete anteriore dell'utero ricopre completamente il canale cervicale, arrivando fino alla parete posteriore dell'utero. La vescica é situata caudalmente. Graduazione della scala : 2 cm per campo

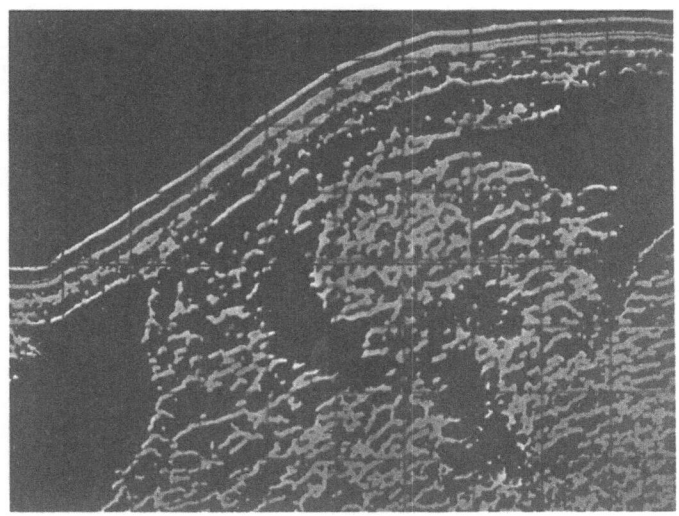

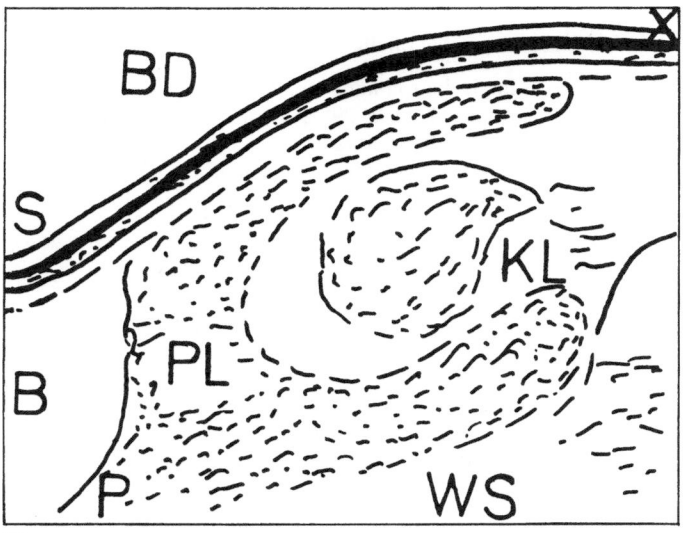

62

Fig. 63. Placenta Praevia Totalis

Longitudinal section in the median line with a placenta praevia totalis in the 29th week. The placenta is inserted on the posterior wall of the uterus. The cervical canal is completely covered by placental tissue

Abb. 63. Placenta praevia totalis

Längsschnitt in der Medianlinie bei einer Placenta praevia totalis in der 29. Woche. Die Placenta inseriert an der Uterushinterwand. Der Cervicalkanal wird vom Placentargewebe völlig überdeckt

Fig. 63. Placenta praevia totalis

Coupe longitudinale dans la ligne médiane. Placenta praevia totalis dans la 29ᵉ semaine. Le placenta s'insère sur la paroi dorsale de l'utérus. La cavité du col utérin est entièrement recouverte par le tissu placentaire

Fig. 63. Placenta previa total. Embarazo de 29 semanas

Corte longitudinal en línea media. Inserción de la placenta en cara posterior. El orificio interno es recubierto totalmente por la placenta

Fig. 63. Placenta previa totale

Sezione longitudinale sulla linea mediana, placenta previa totale nella 29a settimana. La placenta é stavolta localizzata sulla parete posteriore dell'utero. Il canale cervicale é completamente coperto dal tessuto placentare

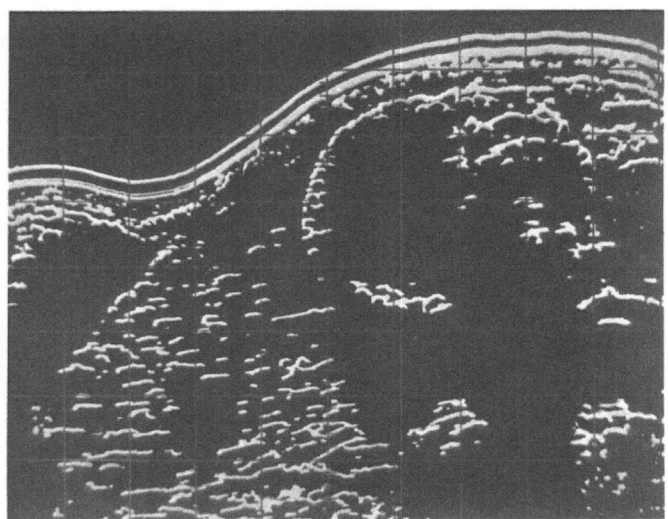

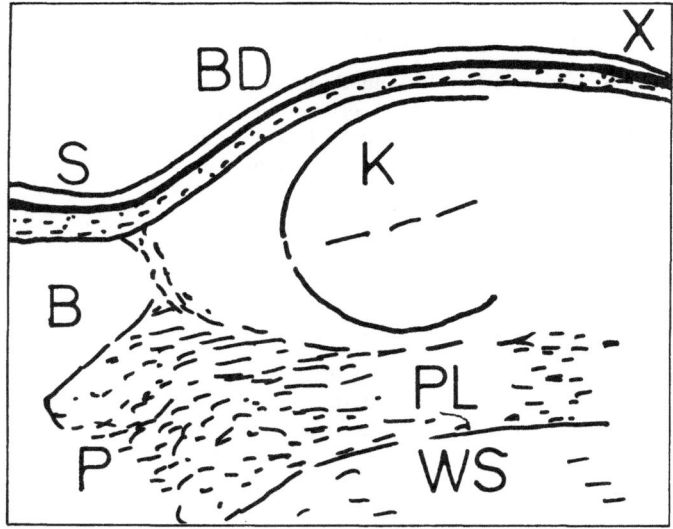

63

Fig. 64. Placenta Praevia Totalis

Cross section at level of symphysis, same case
as Fig. 63. The internal orifice of the uterus is
completely covered with placental tissue. Size
of squares: 2 cm

Abb. 64. Placenta praevia totalis

Querschnitt in Symphysenhöhe, gleicher Fall wie
Abb. 63. Der innere Muttermund ist vollständig
vom Placentargewebe bedeckt. Kantenlänge pro
Feld 2 cm

Fig. 64. Placenta praevia totalis

Coupe transversale à hauteur de la symphyse.
Même cas que l'image 63. L'orifice interne de
l'utérus est complètement recouvert par le tissue
placentaire. Longueur de côté par champ 2 cm

Fig. 64. Placenta previa total

Mismo caso de la figura 63. Corte transversal
a nivel del púbis. El orificio interno es recubierto
totalmente por tejido placentario. 1 división de
escala = 2 cm

Fig. 64. Placenta previa totale

Sezione trasversale all'altezza della sinfisi pubica, caso uguale a quello della Fig. 63. La bocca
uterina interna risulta del tutto coperta da tessuto placentare. Lunghezza del lato: 2 cm per
campo

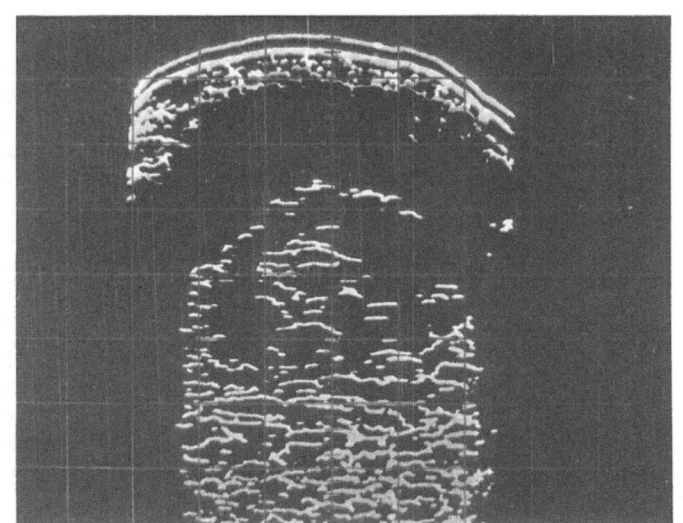

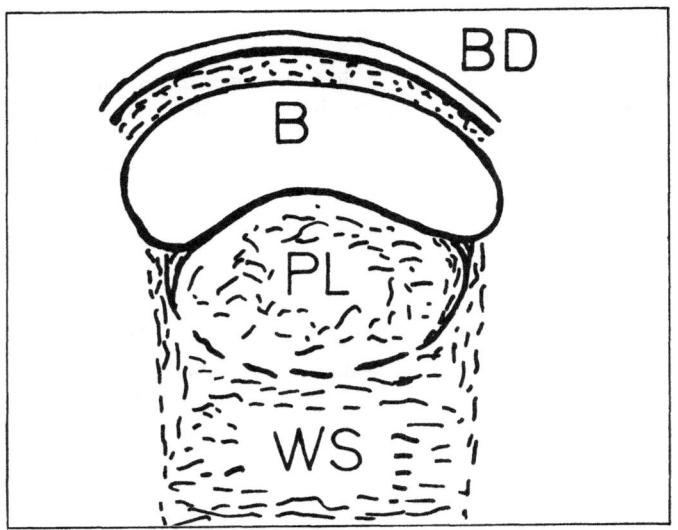

64

Fig. 65. Placenta Praevia Totalis

Longitudinal section in the median line. This is a placenta praevia totalis in the 30th week with breech presentation. Scale division: 2 cm/section

Fig. 66. Placenta Praevia Totalis

Longitudinal section in the median line, same case as Fig. 65. The placenta is located on the posterior wall and completely overlaps the cervical canal. Sharp amnial boundary. Scale divisions: 1 cm/section

Abb. 65. Placenta praevia totalis

Längsschnitt in der Medianlinie. Es handelt sich um eine Placenta praevia totalis in der 30. Woche bei Beckenendlage. Skaleneinteilung pro Feld 2 cm

Abb. 66. Placenta praevia totalis

Längsschnitt in der Medianlinie, gleicher Fall wie Abb. 65. Die Placenta sitzt an der Hinterwand und überlappt den Cervicalkanal völlig. Scharfe amniale Abgrenzung. Skaleneinteilung pro Feld 1 cm

Fig. 65. Placenta praevia totalis

Coupe longitudinale dans la ligne médiane. Il s'agit d'un placenta praevia totalis dans la 30ᵉ semaine, avec présentation par le siège. Graduation par champ 2 cm

Fig. 66. Placenta praevia totalis

Coupe longitudinale dans la ligne médiane. Même cas que l'image 65. Le placenta se trouve à la paroi dorsale et recouvre entièrement la cavité du col utérin. Délimitation amniale marquée. Graduation par champ 1 cm

Fig. 65. Placenta previa total. Podálica

Corte longitudinal en linea media. 1 división de escala = 2 cm

Fig. 66. Placenta previa total

Mismo caso de la figura anterior. Corte longitudinal en línea media. La placenta se encuentra en cara posterior del útero y recubre totalmente el orificio interno 1 división de escala = 1 cm

Fig. 65. Placenta previa totale

Sezione longitudinale sulla linea mediana. Trattasi di placenta previa totale in caso di presentazione podalica nella 30a settimana. Graduazione della scala: 2 cm per campo

Fig. 66. Placenta previa totale

Sezione longitudinale sulla linea mediana, caso uguale a quello della Fig. 65. La placenta risiede sulla parete posteriore e si estende completamente sul canale cervicale. Contorni amniotici ben definiti. Graduazione della scala: 1 cm per campo

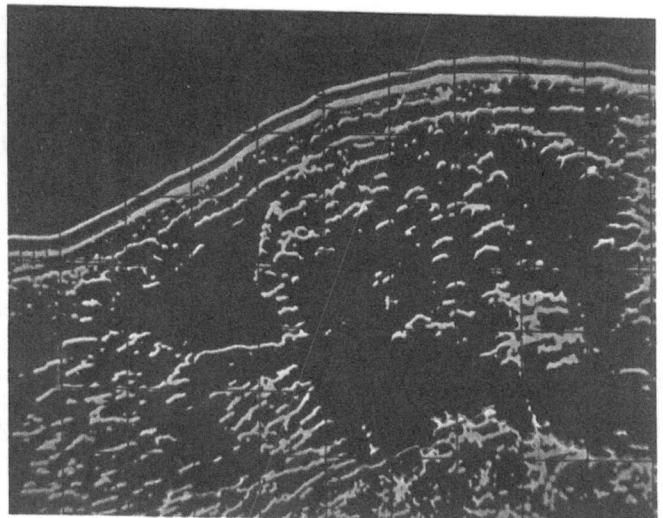

65

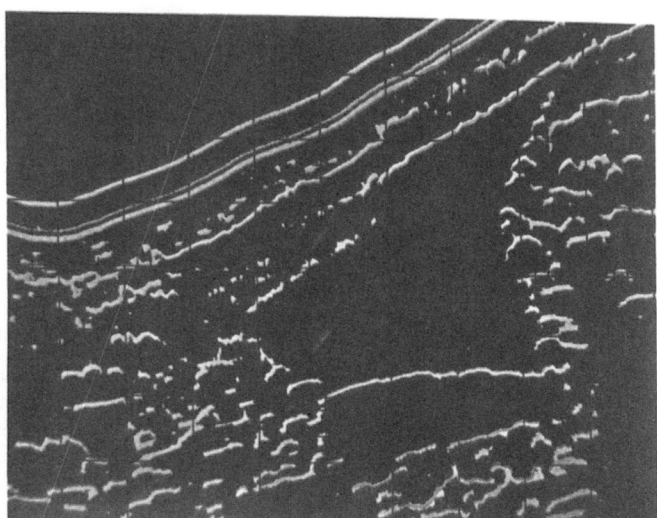

66

Fig. 67. Placenta Praevia Totalis

Longitudinal section in the median line with a placenta praevia totalis in the 35th week. The placenta is in front of the presenting part. The bladder is beyond the placenta

Fig. 68. Placenta Praevia Totalis

Longitudinal section in the median line. The cervical canal is completely covered by the placental tissue. Scale divisions: 2 cm/section. Sound frequency: 2 MHz

Abb. 67. Placenta praevia totalis

Längsschnitt in der Medianlinie bei einer Placenta praevia totalis in der 35. Woche. Die Placenta liegt vor dem vorangehenden Teil. Caudal von der Placenta liegt die Harnblase

Abb. 68. Placenta praevia totalis

Längsschnitt in der Medianlinie. Der Cervicalkanal wird vom Placentargewebe völlig überdeckt. Skaleneinteilung pro Feld 2 cm, Schallfrequenz 2 MHZ

Fig. 67. Placenta praevia totalis

Coupe longitudinale dans la ligne médiane. Placenta praevia totalis dans la 35ᵉ semaine. Le placenta se trouve devant la partie située en avant. Vessie en direction caudale du placenta

Fig. 68. Placenta praevia totalis

Coupe longitudinale dans la ligne médiane. La cavité du col utérin est entièrement recouverte par le tissu placentaire. Graduation par champ 2 cm. Fréquence de son 2 MHz

Fig. 67. Placenta previa total

Corte longitudinal en línea media. Embarazo de 35 semanas. La placenta recubre el orificio interno. Junto a la placenta se encuentra la vejiga

Fig. 68. Placenta previa total

Corte longitudinal en línea media. El orificio interno es recubierto totalmente por la placenta. 1 división de escala = 2 cm. Frecuencia del ultrasonido = 2 MHz

Fig. 67. Placenta previa totale

Sezione longitudinale sulla linea mediana in caso di placenta previa totale nella 35a settimana. La placenta sta davanti alla parte fetale che si impegnerà per prima. Caudalmente alla placenta si vede la vescica urinaria

Fig. 68. Placenta previa totale

Sezione longitudinale sulla linea mediana. Il canale cervicale viene ad essere completamente ricoperto da tessuto placentare. Graduazione della scala: 2 cm per campo. Frequenza: 2 MHZ

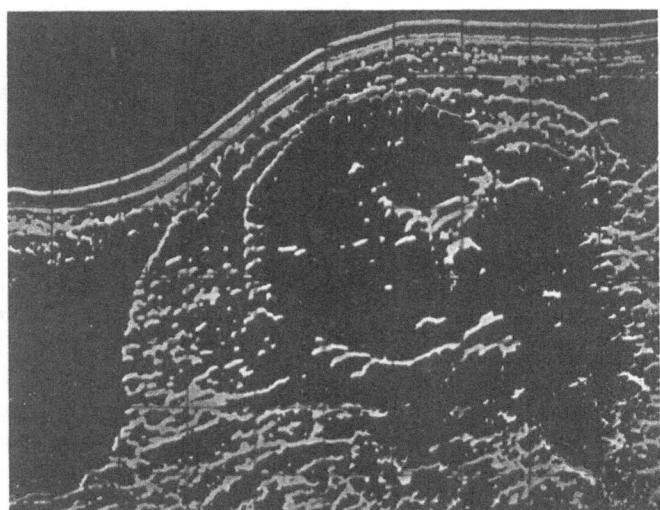

67

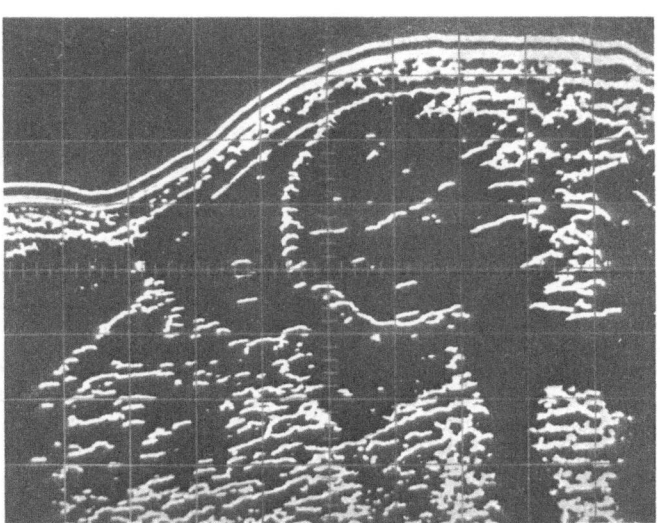

68

Fig. 69. Placenta Praevia Totalis

Longitudinal section in the median line, same case as Fig. 68 with a placenta praevia totalis in the 29th week. Scale divisions: 3 cm/section; sound frequency: 2 MHZ

Fig. 70. Placenta Praevia Totalis

Longitudinal section in the median line. The placenta is located on the anterior wall of the uterus. The placental tissue overlaps the cervical canal and extends to the posterior wall of the uterus

Abb. 69. Placenta praevia totalis

Längsschnitt in der Medianlinie, gleicher Fall wie Abb. 68, bei einer Placenta praevia totalis in der 29. Woche. Skaleneinteilung pro Feld 3 cm, Schallfrequenz 2 MHZ

Abb. 70. Placenta praevia totalis

Längsschnitt in der Medianlinie. Die Placenta sitzt an der Uterusvorderwand. Das Placentargewebe überlappt den Cervicalkanal und reicht bis zur Uterushinterwand

Fig. 69. Placenta praevia totalis

Coupe longitudinale dans la ligne médiane. Même cas que l'image 68. Placenta praevia totalis dans la 29e semaine. Graduation par champ 3 cm. Fréquence de son 2 MHz

Fig. 70. Placenta praevia totalis

Coupe longitudinale dans la ligne médiane. Le placenta se trouve à la paroi ventrale de l'utérus. Le tissu placentaire recouvre la cavité du col utérin et s'étend jusqu'à la paroi dorsale de l'utérus

Fig. 69. Placenta previa total

Mismo caso de la figura 68. Corte longitudinal en línea media. 1 división de escala = 3 cm. Frecuencia del ultrasonido = 2 MHz

Fig. 70. Placenta previa total

Corte longitudinal en línea media. La placenta se encuentra en cara anterior, y recubre el orificio interno y continua en cara posterior

Fig. 69. Placenta previa totale

Sezione longitudinale sulla linea mediana, caso uguale a quello della Fig. 68. Placenta previa totale alla 29a settimana. Graduazione della scala: 3 cm per campo. Frequenza: 2 MHZ

Fig. 70. Placenta previa totale

Sezione longitudinale sulla linea mediana. La placenta risiede sulla parete anteriore dell'utero. Il tessuto placentare arriva al canale cervicale ricoprendolo, e si spinge sino alla parete uterina posteriore

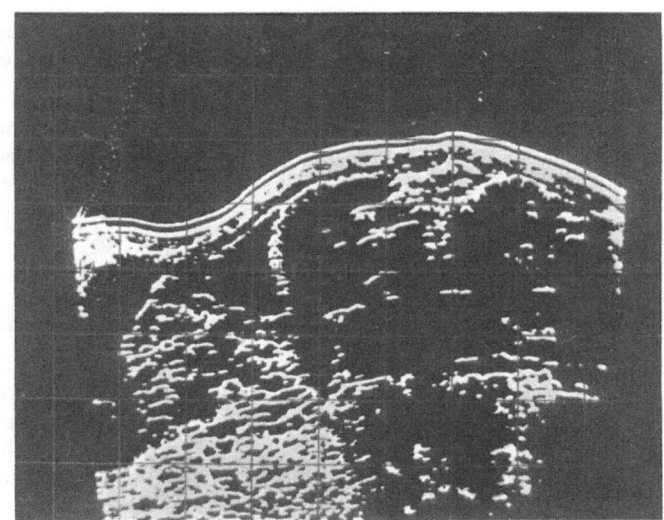

69

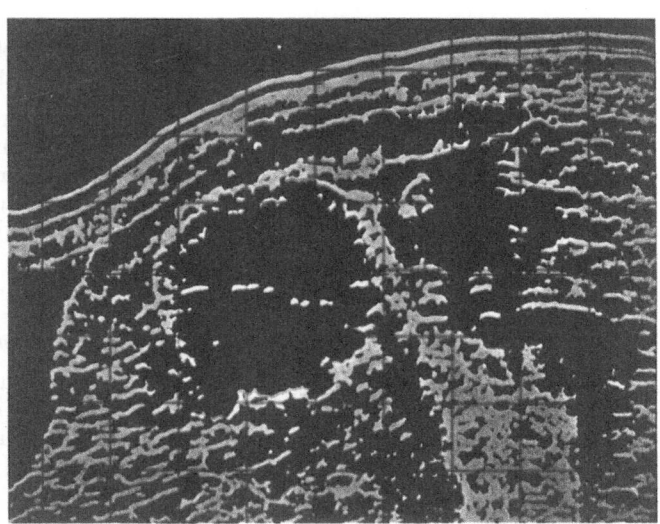

70

Premature Detachment of the Normally Located Placenta

Vorzeitige Lösung der normal sitzenden Placenta
Décollement prématuré du placenta à fixation normale
Desprendimiento prematuro de la placenta normoinserta
Distacco prematuro di placenta

Fig. 71. Premature Detachment of the Normally Located Placenta

Longitudinal section in the median line with total detachment of the normally located placenta. The placenta is detached from the anterior wall of the uterus over its whole area. Scale divisions: 3 cm/section

Abb. 71. Vorzeitige Lösung der normal sitzenden Placenta

Längsschnitt in der Medianlinie bei totaler Ablösung der normal sitzenden Placenta. Die Placenta ist auf ihrer ganzen Fläche von der Uterusvorderwand abgelöst. Skaleneinteilung pro Feld 3 cm

Fig. 71. Décollement prématuré de placenta à fixation normale

Coupe longitudinale dans la ligne médiane en présence d'un décollement total du placenta à fixation normale. Le placenta s'est décollé sur toute sa surface de la paroi ventrale de l'utérus. Graduation par champ 3 cm

Fig. 71. Desprendimiento prematuro de placenta

Corte longitudinal en línea media. La placenta se encuentra totalmente desprendida de la cara anterior del útero. (DPP total). 1 división de escala = 3 cm

Fig. 71. Distacco prematuro di placenta

Sezione longitudinale sulla linea mediana in caso di distacco completo di placenta risiedente in zona del tutto consueta. La placenta si presenta completamente distaccata in tutta la sua superficie dalla parete anteriore dell'utero. Graduazione della scala: 3 cm per campo

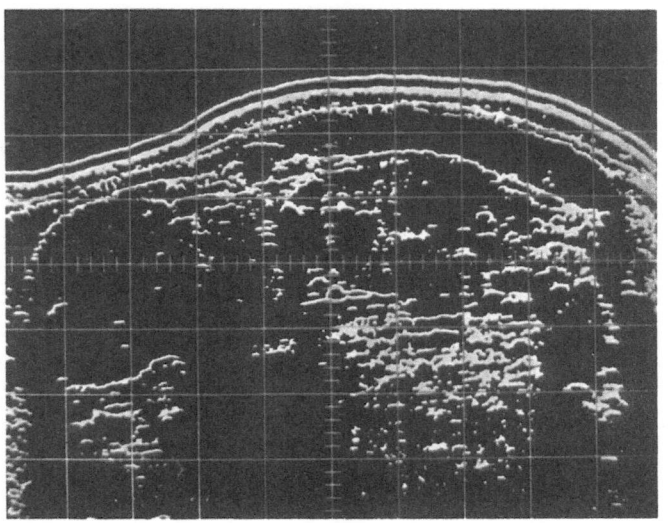

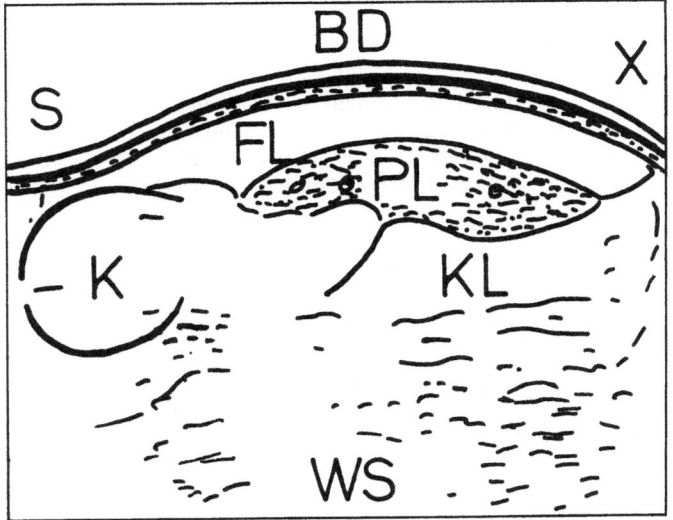

71

Fig. 72. Premature Detachment of the Normally Located Placenta

Longitudinal section in the median line, same case as Fig. 71. Between the anterior wall of the uterus and the placenta there is an echo-free zone 3 cm wide. Scale divisions: 2 cm/section

Abb. 72. Vorzeitige Lösung der normal sitzenden Placenta

Längsschnitt in der Medianlinie, gleicher Fall wie Abb. 71. Zwischen Uterusvorderwand und Placenta besteht eine echofreie Zone von 3 cm Breite. Skaleneinteilung pro Feld 2 cm

Fig. 72. Décollement prématuré de placenta à fixation normale

Coupe longitudinale dans la ligne médiane, même cas que l'image 71. Entre la paroi ventrale de l'utérus et le placenta il existe une zone exempte d'échos de 3 cm de large. Graduation par champ 2 cm

Fig. 72. Desprendimiento prematuro de placenta

Mismo caso de la figura 71. Corte longitudinal en línea media. Entre cara anterior del útero y placenta se encuentra una zona libre de ecos de 3 cm de ancho. 1 división de escala = 2 cm

Fig. 72. Distacco prematuro di placenta

Sezione longitudinale sulla linea mediana, caso uguale a quello della Fig. 71. Tra la parete uterina anteriore e la placenta c'é una zona di 3 cm di ampiezza priva di eco. Graduazione della scala: 2 cm per campo

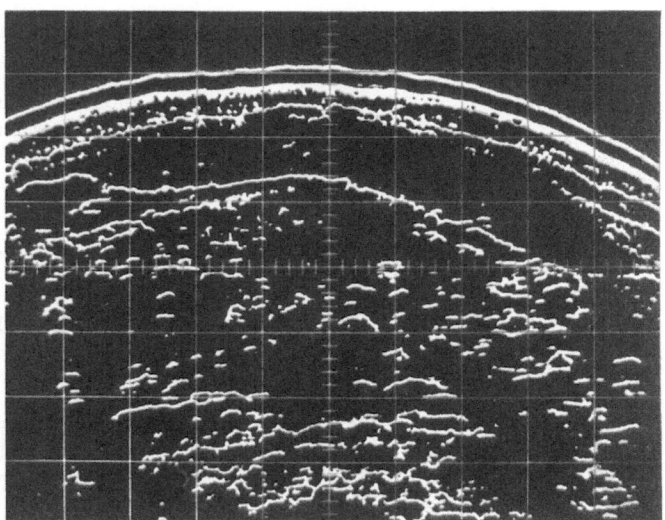

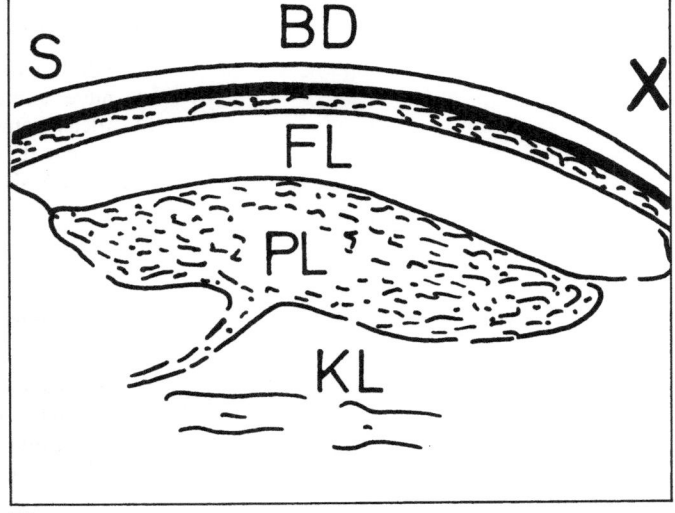

72

Twins

Zwillinge
Jumeaux
Embrazo gemelar
Gemelli

Fig. 73. Twin Pregnancy in the 27th Week

Longitudinal section in the median line of the mother. Twins in vertex presentation, both biparietal diameters are 6.4 cm; sides of squares 3 cm long. Sound frequency 2.5 MHz

Abb. 73. Zwillingsschwangerschaft in der 27. Woche

Längsschnitt in der Medianlinie der Mutter, Zwillinge in Kopflage, beide biparietalen Durchmesser betragen 6,4 cm, Kantenlänge pro Feld 3 cm. Schallfrequenz 2,5 MHZ

Fig. 73. Grossesse gémellaire dans la 27e semaine

Coupe longitudinale dans la ligne médiane de la mère. Jumeaux en présentation céphalique. Les deux diamètres bipariétaux mesurent 6,4 cm. Longueur de côté par champ 3 cm. Fréquence de son 2,5 MHz

Fig. 73. Embarazo gemelar — 27 semanas de gestación

Corte longitudinal en línea media. Ambos fetos en cefálica. Diámetro biparietal en ambos: 6,4 cm. 1 división de escala = 3 cm. Frecuencia del ultrasonido = 2,5 MHz

Fig. 73. Gravidanza gemellare nella 27a settimana

Sezione longitudinale nella linea mediana. Gemelli in posizione cefalica, i due diametri biparietali arrivano a 6,4 cm, lunghezza del lato: 3 cm. per campo. Frequenza: 2,5 MHZ

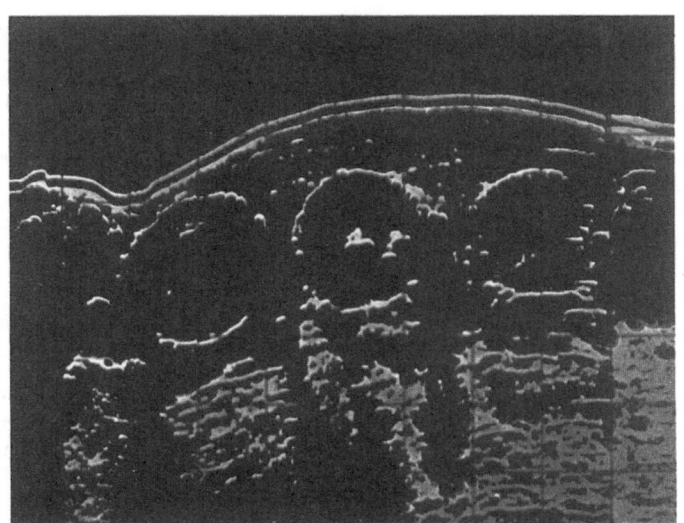

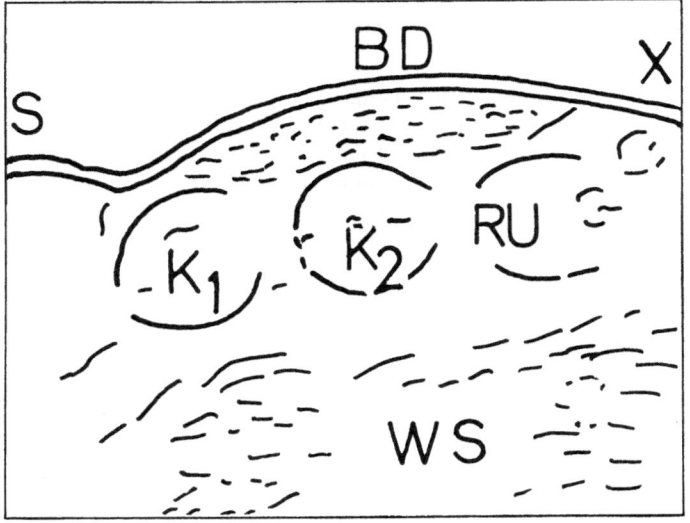

73

Fig. 74. Hydramnios and Twins in the 23rd Week

Longitudinal section in the median line, twins in head presentation. Surrounding them are extensive homogeneous echo-free regions, which correspond to the amniotic fluid. Torso and small parts visible beside the heads. Placenta is on the posterior wall

Fig. 75. Twin Pregnancy in the 30th Week

Longitudinal section in the median line, twins in head presentation; biparietal diameter in both fetuses 7.2 cm; length of sides of squares 3 cm. Sound frequency 2 MHz

Abb. 74. Hydramnion und Zwillinge in der 23. Woche

Längsschnitt in der Medianlinie, Zwillinge in Kopflage. In der Umgebung ausgedehnte homogene echofreie Bezirke, welche der Amnionflüssigkeit entsprechen. Neben den Köpfen Rumpf und kleine Teile sichtbar. Placenta liegt an der Hinterwand

Abb. 75. Zwillingsschwangerschaft in der 30. Woche

Längsschnitt in der Medianlinie, Zwillinge in Kopflage, biparietaler DM bei beiden Kindern 7,2 cm, Kantenlänge pro Feld 3 cm. Schallfrequenz 2 MHZ

Fig. 74. Hydramnios et jumeaux dans la 23e semaine

Coupe longitudinale dans la ligne médiane. Jumeaux en présentation céphalique. Dans le voisinage, des zones étendues exemptes d'échos se rapportant au liquide amniotique. Le tronc et des parties foetales sont visibles à côté des têtes. Le placenta se trouve à la paroi dorsale

Fig. 75. Grossesse gémellaire dans la 30e semaine

Coupe longitudinale dans la ligne médiane. Jumeaux en présentation céphalique. Diamètre biparétal des deux enfants: 7,2 cm. Longueur de côté par champ 3 cm. Fréquence de son 2 MHz

Fig. 74. Embarazo gemelar e hidramnios — 23 semanas de gestación

Corte longitudinal en línea media. Ambos gemelos en cefálica. La zona libre de ecos corresponde al líquido amniótico. Se pueden observar las 2 cabezas, cuerpo y extremidades fetales. La placenta está inserta en la cara posterior del útero

Fig. 75. Embarazo gemelar — 30 semanas de gestación

Corte longitudinal en línea media. Ambos gemelos en cefálica. Diámetro biparietal en ambos: 7,2 cm. 1 división de escala = 3 cm. Frecuencia del ultrasonido = 2 MHz

Fig. 74. Idramnio e gemelli nella 23a settimana

Sezione longitudinale sulla linea mediana, gemelli in presentazione cefalica. Si noti una zona abbastanza estesa priva di eco, corrispondente alla zona occupata dal liquido amniotico. In vicinanza delle teste fetali sono visibili torace e estremità. La placenta é nella parete posteriore

Fig. 75. Gravidanza gemellare nell 30a settimana

Sezione longitudinale sulla linea mediana, gemelli in presentazione cefalica, diametro biparietale dei due bambini: 7,2 cm, lunghezza del lato per campo: 3 cm. Frequenza: 2 MHZ

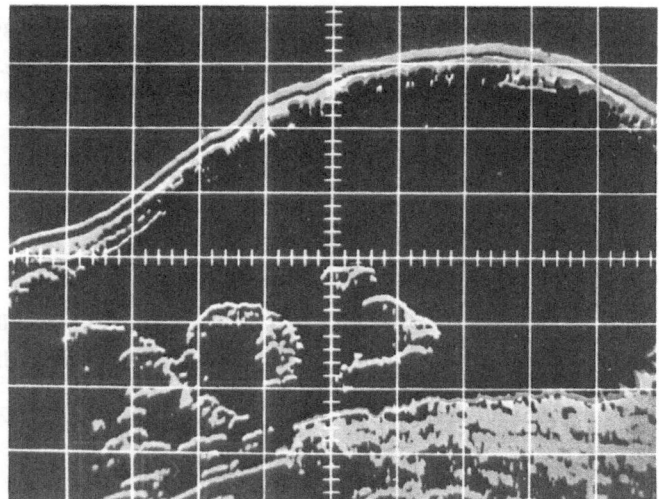

74

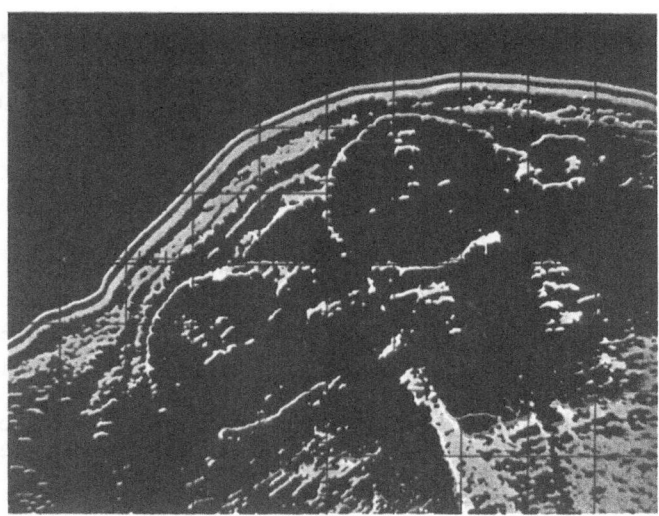

75

Fig. 76. Pregnancy in the 25th Week

Longitudinal section in the median line, twins in head presentation; biparietal diameter of both fetuses 5.8 cm, sides of squares 3 cm long. Sound frequency 2 MHz

Fig. 77. Longitudinal Section in the Median Line

Same case as Fig. 76, both heads side by side. Grid divisions 2 cm, sound frequency 2 MHz

Abb. 76. Schwangerschaft in der 25. Woche

Längsschnitt in der Medianlinie, Zwillinge in Kopflage, biparietaler DM bei beiden Kindern 5,8 cm, Kantenlänge pro Feld 3 cm. Schallfrequenz 2 MHZ

Abb. 77. Längsschnitt in der Medianlinie

Gleicher Fall wie Abb. 76, beide Köpfe nebeneinander, Rastereinteilung 2 cm, Schallfrequenz 2 MHZ

Fig. 76. Grossesse dans la 25ᵉ semaine

Coupe longitudinale dans la ligne médiane. Jumeaux en présentation céphalique. Diamètre bipariétal des deux enfants: 5,8 cm. Longueur de côté par champ 3 cm. Fréquence de son 2 MHz

Fig. 77. Coupe longitudinale dans la ligne médiane

Même cas que l'image 76. Les deux têtes sont côte à côte. Quadrillage: 2 cm. Fréquence de son 2 MHz

Fig. 76. Embarazo gemelar — 25 semanas de gestación

Corte longitudinal en línea media. Ambos fetos en cefálica, con diámetro biparietal de 5,8 cm. 1 división de escala = 3 cm. Frecuencia del ultrasonido = 2 MHz

Fig. 77. Embarazo gemelar

Mismo caso de la figura anterior. Corte longitudinal en línea media. Se pueden observar ambos polos cefálicos. 1 división de escala = 2 cm. Frecuencia del ultrasonido = 2 MHz

Fig. 76. Gravidanza nella 25a settimana

Sezione longitudinale sulla linea mediana, gemelli in presentazione cefalica, diametro biparietale dei due bambini: 5,8 cm. lunghezza del lato 3 cm per campo. Frequenza: 2 MHZ

Fig. 77. Sezione longitudinale sulla linea mediana

Caso uguale alla figura 76. Le due teste sono una accanto all' altra. Frequenza: 2 MHZ

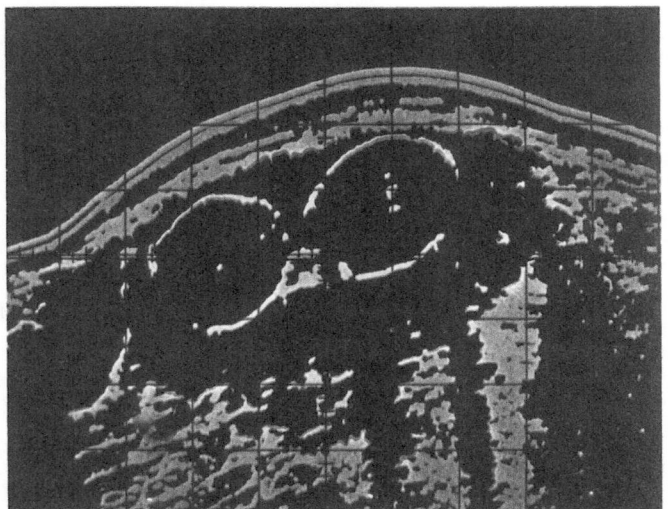

76

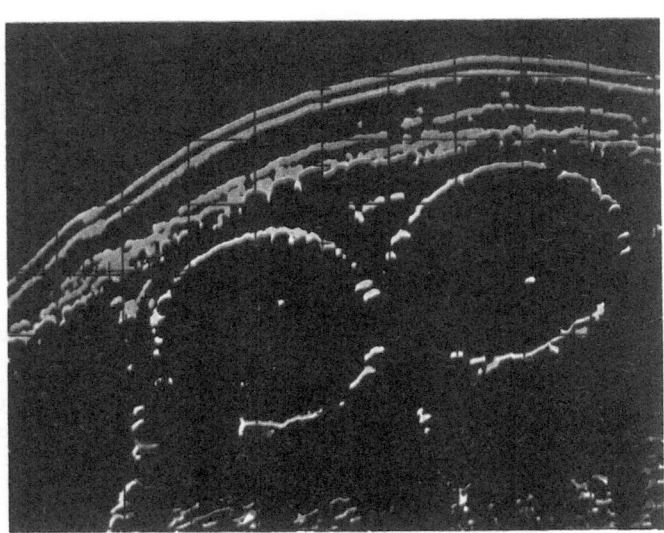

77

Fig. 78. Twin Pregnancy in the 30th Week

Longitudinal section in the median line, same case as Fig. 75, but here the length of the sides of the squares is 3 cm

Fig. 79. Twin Pregnancy in the 30th Week

Longitudinal section in the median line in the same case as Fig. 75. Side of squares here 3 cm

Abb. 78. Zwillingsschwangerschaft in der 30. Woche

Längsschnitt in der Medianlinie, gleicher Fall wie Abb. 75, hier beträgt die Kantenlänge pro Feld 3 cm

Abb. 79. Zwillingsschwangerschaft in der 30. Woche

Längsschnitt in der Medianlinie bei gleichem Fall wie 75. Kantenlänge beträgt hier 3 cm

Fig. 78. Grossesse gémallaire dans la 30ᵉ semaine

Coupe longitudinale dans la ligne médiane. Même cas que image 75. La longueur de côté est ici de 3 cm

Fig. 79. Grossesse gémellaire dans la 30ᵉ semaine

Coupe longitudinale dans la ligne médiane. Même cas que l'image 75. Longueur de côté 3 cm

Fig. 78. Embarazo gemelar

Mismo caso de la figura 75, pero con 30 semanas de gestación. Corte longitudinal en línea media. 1 división de escala = 3 cm

Fig. 79. Embarazo gemelar

Mismo caso de la figura 75, pero con 30 semanas de gestación. Corte longitudinal en línea media. 1 división de escala = 3 cm

Fig. 78. Gravidanza gemellare nella 30a settimana

Sezione longitudinale sulla linea mediana, caso uguale a quello della Fig. 75. In questa .nuova figura la lunghezza del lato arriva a 3 cm

Fig. 79. Gravidanza gemellare nella 30a settimana

Sezione longitudinale sulla linea mediana, caso uguale a quello illustrato nella Fig. 75. Lunghezza del lato: 3 cm

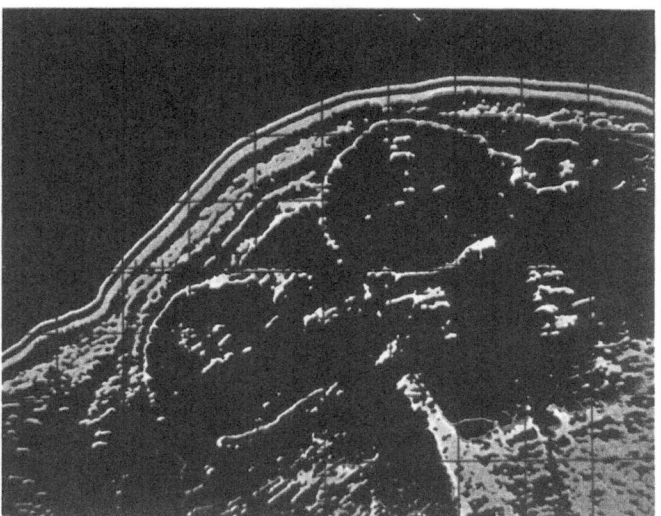

78

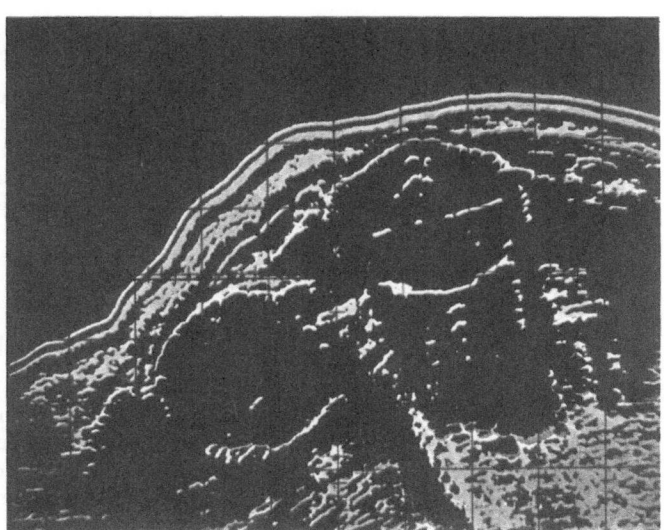

79

Vesicular Moles

Blasenmole
Môle hydatiforme
Mola hidatídica
Mola vescicolare

Fig. 80. Vesicular Mole in the 19th Week

Suprapubic cross section of a vesicular mole in the 19th week. The whole cavity is full of "dot-and-dash"-like echos, which mostly correspond to the cyst wall. Sides of squares are 2 cm long

Abb. 80. Blasenmole in der 19. Woche

Suprasymphysärer Querschnitt einer Blasenmole in der 19. Woche. Ganzes Cavum ist voll von punkt- und strichförmigen Echos, die zum großen Teil der Cystenwand entsprechen. Kantenlänge pro Feld 2 cm

Fig. 80. Môle hydatiforme dans la 19ᵉ semaine

Coupe transversale suprasymphysaire d'une môle hydatiforme dans la 19ᵉ semaine. Toute la cavité est remplie d'échos en forme de points et de traits, se rapportant en majeure partie à la paroi du kyste. Longueur de côté par champ 2 cm

Fig. 80. Mola hidatídica—19 semanas de amenorrea

Corte transversal suprapúbico. Toda la cavidad uterina aparece con ecos puntiformes o lineares debido a las delimitaciones de las vesículas. 1 división de escala = 2 cm

Fig. 80. Mola vescicolare nella 19a settimana

Sezione soprasinfisaria di mola vescicolare nella 19a settimana di gravidanza. La cavità uterina é completamente occupata da echi puntiformi e echi a forma di linea. Lunghezza del lato: 2 cm per campo

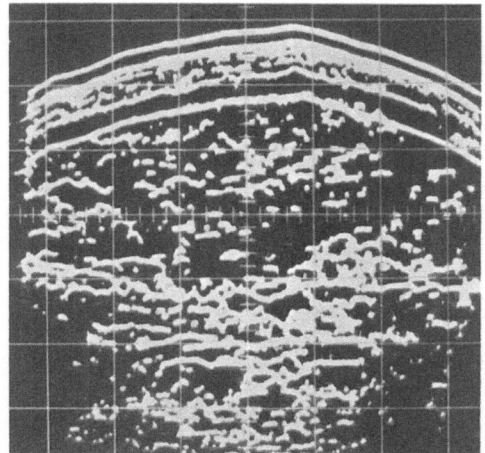
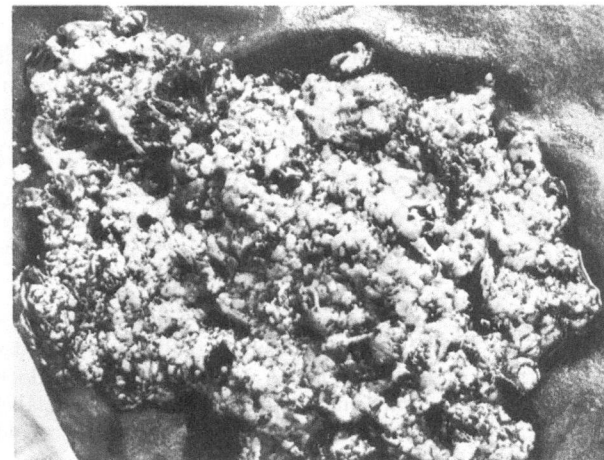

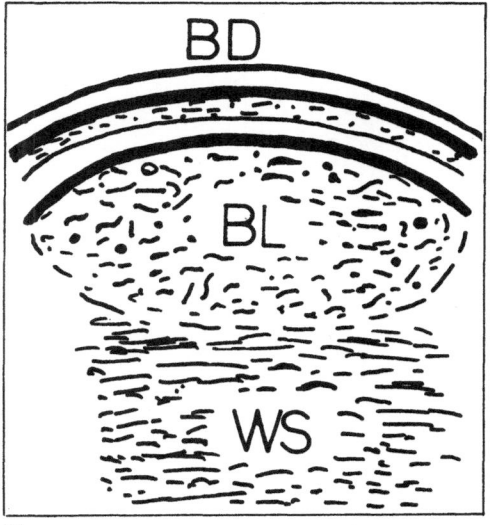

80

Fig. 81. Vesicular Mole in the 19th Week

Ultrasonic echogram of a vesicular mole in the 19th week. Same case as Fig. 80, but in longitudinal section, from the navel toward the symphysis

Abb. 81. Blasenmole in der 19. Woche

Ultraschallechogramm einer Blasenmole in der 19. Woche. Gleicher Fall wie Abb. 80, jedoch im longitudinalen Schnitt, und zwar vom Nabel Richtung Symphyse. Skaleneinteilung pro Feld 2 cm

Fig. 81. Môle hydatiforme dans la 19ᵉ semaine

Echogramme à ultrasons d'une môle hydatiforme dans la 19ᵉ semaine. Même cas que l'image 80. mais en coupe longitudinale, notamment du nombril vers la symphyse. Graduation par champ 2 cm

Fig. 81. Mola hidatídica

Mismo caso de la figura 80. Corte longitudinal en línea media infraumbilical. 1 división de escala = 2 cm

Fig. 81. Mola vescicolare nella 19a settimana

Caso eguale alla Fig. 80. Questa volta pero' in sezione longitudinale dall'ombelico verso la sinfisi pubica. Graduazione della scala: 2 cm per campo

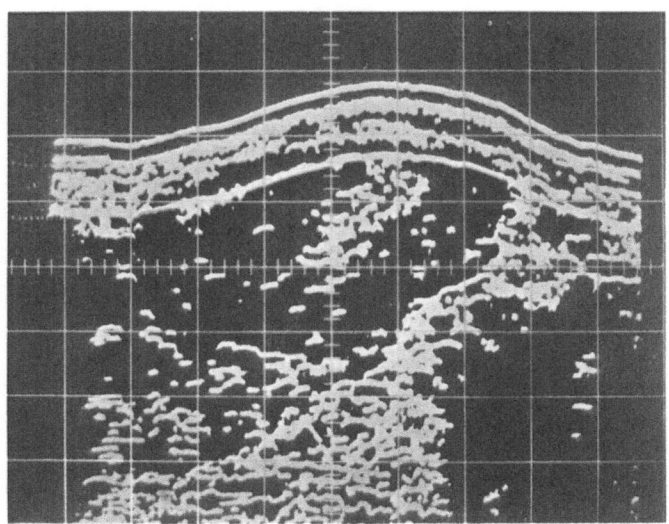

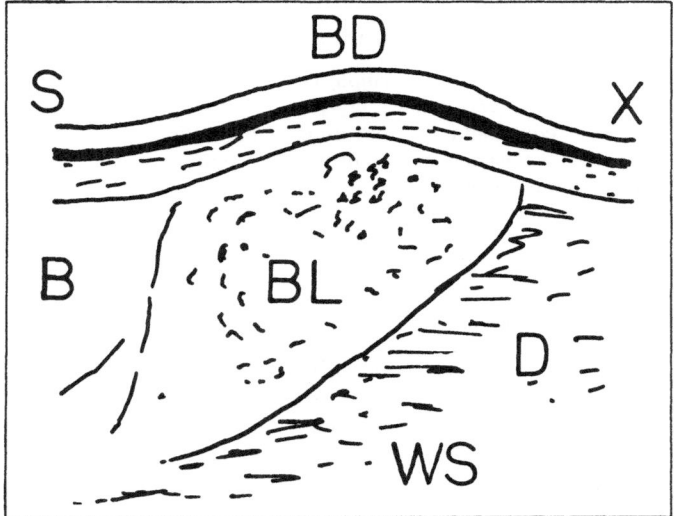

81

Fig. 82. Partial Vesicular Mole

Suprapubic cross section in the case of an amenorrhoea of 20 weeks.
In the cavity there was a severely deformed and macerated fetus and also partly cystically denatured chorionic villi, with an anterior-wall placenta

Abb. 82. Partielle Blasenmole

Suprasymphysärer Querschnitt bei einer Amenorrhoe von 20 Wochen.
Im Cavum fanden sich ein stark deformierter und macerierter Fetus sowie z.T. blasig entartete Chorionzotten bei Vorderwandplacenta

Fig. 82. Môle hydatiforme partielle

Coupe transversale suprasymphysaire après une aménorrhée de 20 semaines.
La cavité contenait un foetus fortement déformé et macéré, ainsi que des villosités placentaires présentant partiellement une dégénérescence vésiculeuse. Placenta ventral

Fig. 82. Mola hidatídica parcial

Corte transversal suprapúbico. 20 semanas de amenorrea. En la cavidad uterina se encuentra un feto deformado y macerado, asi como también vesículas de las vellosidades coriónicas de la placenta (inserción en cara anterior del útero)

Fig. 82. Mola vescicolare parziale

Sezione soprasinfisaria in caso di amenorrea di 20 settimane. Nella cavità uterina si trova un feto fortemente deformato e macerato, e villi coriali in parziale degenerazione vescicolare. La placenta si trova sulla parete anteriore

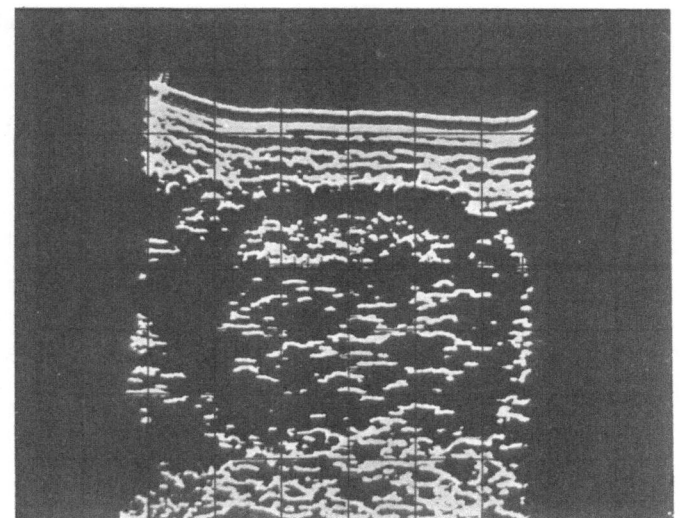

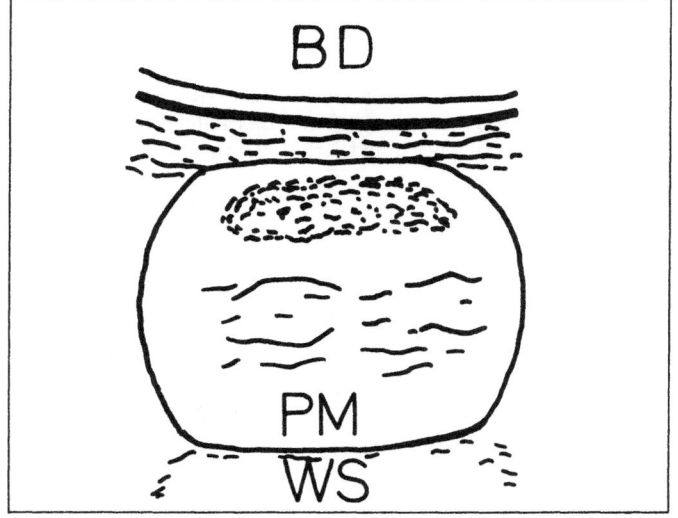

82

Fig. 83. Vesicular Mole in the 16th Week

Ultrasonic echogram of a vesicular mole in the 16th week, suprapubic cross section with scale divisions of 2 cm. The whole cavum gives the effect of a picture in a snowstorm (vesicular mole)

Fig. 84. Vesicular Mole in the 16th Week

Longitudinal section in the center-line. Same case as Fig. 83, no fetal parts detectable. The urinary bladder is beyond the uterus

Abb. 83. Blasenmole in der 16. Woche

Ultraschallechogramm einer Blasenmole in der 16. Woche, suprapubischer Querschnitt mit Skaleneinteilung von 2 cm. Das ganze Cavum wirkt wie ein Bild mit Schneegestöber (Blasenmole)

Abb. 84. Blasenmole in der 16. Woche

Longitudinaler Schnitt in der Mittellinie. Gleicher Fall wie Abb. 83, keine fetalen Elemente nachweisbar. Caudal vom Uterus liegt die Harnblase

Fig. 83. Môle hydatiforme dans la 16ᵉ semaine

Echogramme à ultrasons d'une môle hydatiforme dans la 16ᵉ semaine. Coupe transversale suprapubienne avec graduation de 2 cm. La cavité entière prend l'apparence d'un tourbillon de neige (môle hydatiforme)

Fig. 84. Môle hydatiforme dans la 16ᵉ semaine

Coupe longitudinale dans la ligne médiane. Même cas que l'image 83. Pas d'éléments foetaux perceptibles. La vessie se trouve en direction caudale de l'utérus

Fig. 83. Mola hidatídica — 16 semanas de amenorrea

Corte transversal suprapúbico. La imagen dentro de la cadidad uterina se parece a copos de nieve (mola). 1 división de escala = 2 cm

Fig. 84. Mola hidatídica

Mismo caso de la figura anterior. Corte longitudinal. No se pueden observar estructuras fetales. Vecino al útero, en dirección caudal, se encuentra la vejiga

Fig. 83. Mola vescicolare nella 16a settimana

Ecogramma di una mola vescicolare nella sedicesima settimana, sezione soprapubica; graduazione di scala di 2 cm. La cavità uterina presenta il quadro tipico della cosidetta "tempesta di neve" (mola vescicolare)

Fig. 84. Mola vescicolare nella sedicesima settimana

Sezione longitudinale sulla linea mediana, caso uguale alla Fig. 83, parti fetali non visibili. Caudalmente all'utero é situata la vescica urinaria

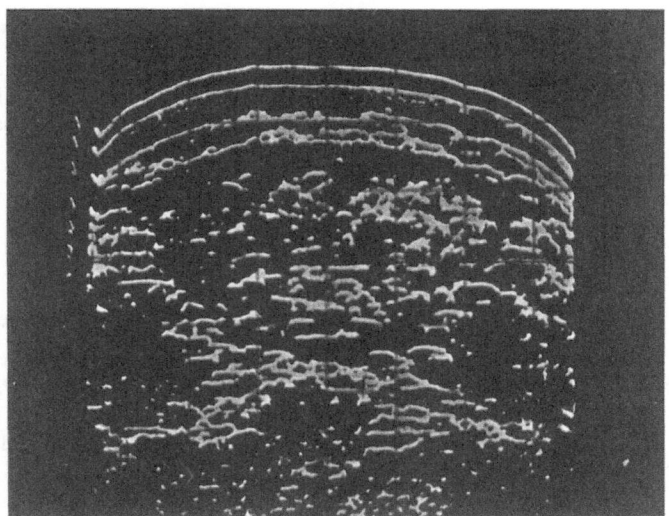

83

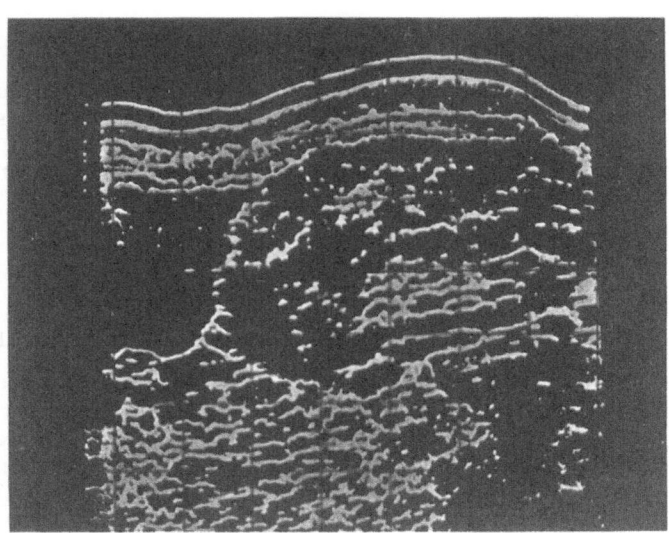

84

Fig. 85. Vesicular Mole in the 20th Week

Suprapubic cross section with a vesicular mole in the 20th week. Here again, the whole cavity is filled with dot-and-dash echos; no fetal parts are recognisable

Fig. 86. Vesicular Mole in the 20th Week

Longitudinal section from the navel toward the symphysis in the same patient as Fig. 85. Urinary bladder lies beyond the uterus. Scale divisions: 2 cm section

Abb. 85. Blasenmole in der 20. Woche

Querschnitt suprapubisch bei einer Blasenmole in der 20. Woche. Hier ist ebenfalls das ganze Cavum mit punkt- und strichförmigen Echos gefüllt, keine fetalen Teile erkennbar

Abb. 86. Blasenmole in der 20. Woche

Längsschnitt vom Nabel Richtung Symphyse bei der gleichen Patientin wie Abb. 85. Caudal vom Uterus liegt die Harnblase. Skaleneinteilung 2 cm pro Feld

Fig. 85. Môle hydatiforme dans la 20ᵉ semaine

Coupe transversale suprapubienne d'une môle hydatiforme dans la 20ᵉ semaine. Ici également, la cavité entière est remplie d'échos en forme de points et de traits. Pas de parties foetales perceptibles

Fig. 86. Môle hydatiforme dans la 20ᵉ semaine

Coupe longitudinale, du nombril en direction de la symphyse, de la même patiente que celle de l'image 85. La vessie se trouve en direction caudale de l'utérus. Graduation 2 cm par champ

Fig. 85. Mola hidatídica — 20 semanas de amenorrea

Corte transversal suprapúbico. Toda la cavidad uterina aparece con ecos puntiformes y lineares. No se pueden ver estructuras fetales

Fig. 86. Mola hidatiforme

Mismo caso de la figura anterior. Corte longitudinal en línea media infraumbilical. Vecino al útero, en dirección caudal, se encuentra la vejiga. 1 división de escala = 2 cm

Fig. 85. Mola vescicolare nella 20a settimana

Sezione soprapubica in caso di mola vescicolare nella 20a settimana. Anche qui la cavità uterina é occupata da echi puntiformi e lineari, parti fetali non riconoscibili

Fig. 86. Mola vescicolare nella 20a settimana

Sezione longitudinale in partenza dall'ombelico in direzione della sinfisi pubica, caso eguale alla Fig. 85 (stessa paziente). Caudalmente all'utero la vescica urinaria. Graduazione di scala: 2 cm per campo

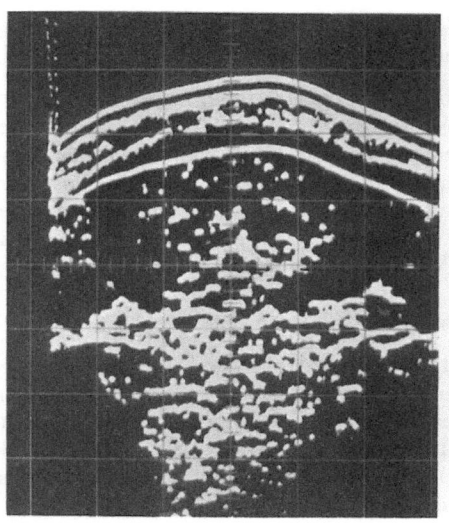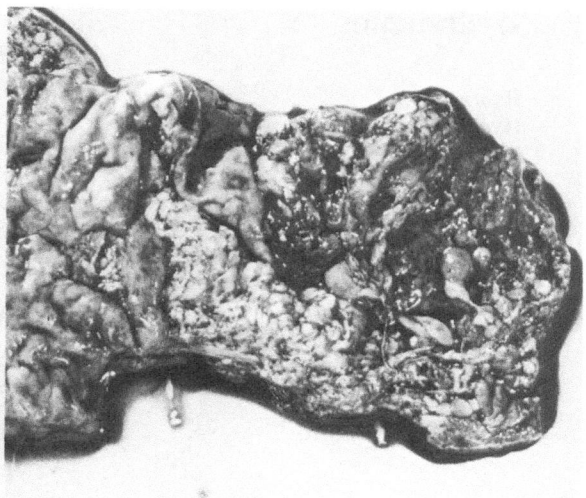

85

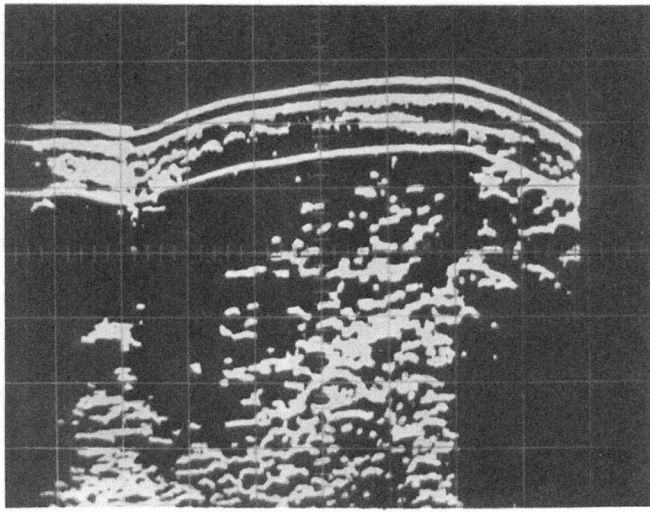

86

Hydramnios

Hydramnion
Hydramnios
Hidramnios
Idramnio

Fig. 87. Hydramnios in the 37th Week of Pregnancy

Longitudinal section in the median line. The fetus is surrounded by a wide, echo-free, homogeneous region, which corresponds to the amniotic fluid. Biparietal diameter is 9.3 cm. Posteriorwall placenta (also confirmed manually). Sides of squares are 3 cm long. Sound frequency is 2 MHz

Abb. 87. Hydramnion in der 37. Woche

Längsschnitt in der Medianlinie. Fetus ist umgeben von einem breiten, echofreien, homogenen Bezirk, der der Amnionflüssigkeit entspricht. Biparietaler DM beträgt 9,3 cm, Hinterwandplacenta (auch manuell bestätigt). Kantenlänge pro Feld 3 cm. Schallfrequenz 2 MHZ

Fig. 87. Hydramnios dans la 37ᵉ semaine de grossesse

Coupe longitudinale dans la ligne médiane. Le foetus est entouré d'une large zone, exempte d'échos et homogène qui correspond au liquide amniotique. Le diamètre bipariétal mesure 9,3 cm. Placenta dorsal (constaté aussi manuellement). Longueur de côté par champ 3 cm. Fréquence de son 2 MHz

Fig. 87. Hidramnios — Embarazo de 37 semanas de gestación

Corte longitudinal en línea medial. El feto se encuentra rodeado por una extensa zona homogénea libre de ecos, que corresponde al líquido amniótico. El diámetro biparietal es de 9,3 cm. Localización de la placenta en cara posterior del útero. 1 división de escala = 3 cm. Frecuencia del ultrasonido = 2 MHz

Fig. 87. Idramnio nella 37a settimana di gravidanza

Sezione longitudinale sulla linea mediana. Il feto é circondato da un ampia zona omegenea e priva di eco, che corrisponde alla zona occupata dal liquido amniotico. Il diametro biparietale é di 9,3 cm. La placenta é sulla parete posteriore uterina (reporto confermato anche manualmente) Lunghezza del lato 3 cm per campo, frequenza: 2 MHZ

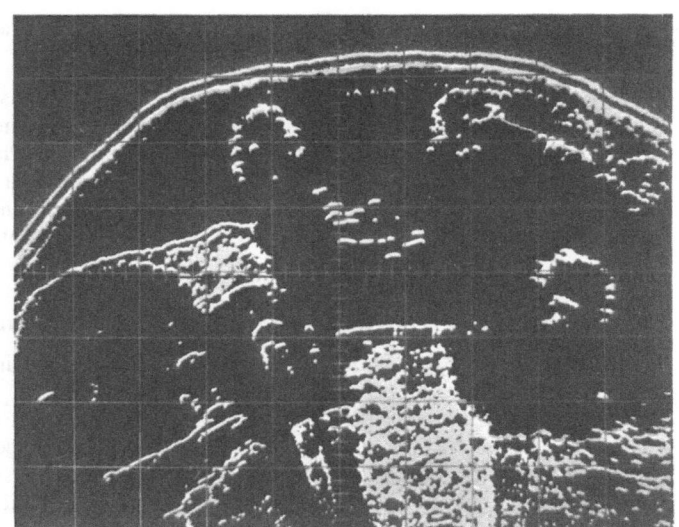

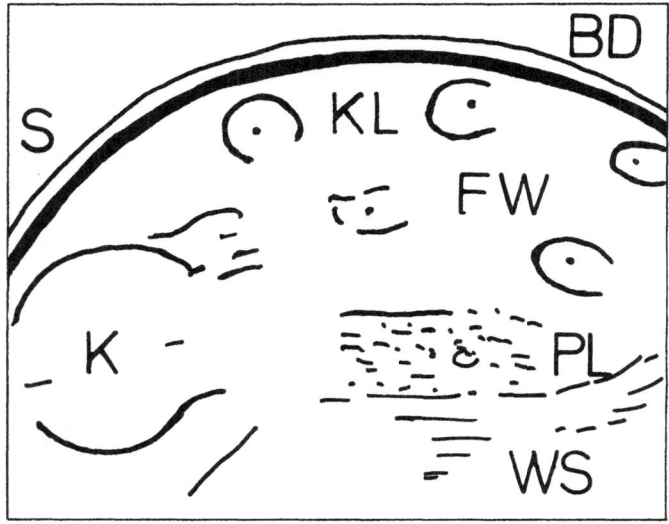

87

Fig. 88. Hydramnios in the 40th Week of Pregnancy

Longitudinal section in the median line, fetus again in an echo-free region. Biparietal diameter is 9.6 cm; placenta is located on the posterior wall. Amniotic fluid: 5 liters—confirmed by operation. (Hydramnios was caused by oesophagus atresia in the fetus)

Abb. 88. Hydramnion in der 40. Woche

Längsschnitt in der Medianlinie, wiederum Fetus in einem echofreien Bezirk. Biparietaler DM beträgt 9,6 cm, Placenta liegt an der Hinterwand, Fruchtwasser 5 l (operativ bestätigt; Hydramnion war bedingt durch Oesophagusatresie des Kindes)

Fig. 88. Hydramnios dans la 40ᵉ semaine de grossesse

Coupe longitudinale dans la ligne médiane. Le foetus se trouve à nouveau dans une zone exempte d'échos. Le diamètre bipariétal mesure 9,6 cm. Le placenta se trouve à la paroi dorsale. Liquide amniotique 5 litres. (Confirmé par voie opératoire. L'hydramnios était déterminé par une atrésie de l'oesophage de l'enfant)

Fig. 88. Hidramnios. Embarazo de 40 semanas de gestación

Corte longitudinal en línea media. El feto se encuentra rodeado de una zona libre de ecos. Diámetro biparietal: 9,6 cm. Inserción de la placenta en cara posterior del útero. Cantidad de líquido amniótico: 5 litros, verificados durante la intervención quirúrgica. Causa del hidramnios: atresia del esófago

Fig. 88. Idramnio nella 40a settimana di gravidanza

Sezione longitudinale sulla linea mediana, il feto si trova di nuovo in un ampia zona priva di eco. Diametro biparietale 9,6 cm, la placenta risiede sulla parete posteriore, quantità del liquido amniotico: 5 litri. (Quantità confermata anche in sede operatoria). L'idramnio era in questo caso causato da un'atresia esofagea del bambino

Fig. 89. Hydramnios in the 37th Week of pregnancy

Longitudinal section in the median line, amniotic fluid volume approx. 3 liters, biparietal diameter 9.3 cm. Placenta is located on the posterior wall with clear strip-shaped echos, which correspond to the amniotic boundary. Small parts are visible in front of the placenta

Abb. 89. Hydramnion in der 37. Woche

Längsschnitt in der Medianlinie, Fruchtwassermenge ca 3 l, biparietaler DM beträgt 9,3 cm. Placenta liegt an der Hinterwand mit deutlich streifenförmigen Echos, die der amnialen Begrenzung entsprechen. Vor der Placenta sind kleine Teile sichtbar

Fig. 89. Hydramnios dans la 37ᵉ semaine de grossesse

Coupe longitudinale dans la ligne médiane. Quantité de liquide amniotique: 3 l. Le diamètre bipariétal mesure 9,3 cm. Le placenta se trouve à la paroi dorsale et présente des échos en forme de traits bien distincts, correspondant à la délimitation amniale. Devant le placenta on aperçoit des parties foetales

Fig. 89. Hidramnios — Embarazo de 37 semanas de gestación

Corte longitudinal en línea media. Cantidad de líquido amniótico: aprox. 3 litros. Diámetro biparietal: 9,3 cm. La placenta se encuentra en cara posterior del útero, delante de ella se encuentran extremidades fetales

Fig. 89. Idramnio nella 37a settimana di gravidanza

Sezione longitudinale sulla linea mediana; quantità del liquido amniotico: 3 litri, diametro biparietale: 9,3 cm. La placenta é sulla parete posteriore (l'eco é visibile chiaramente sotto forma lineare). Davanti alla placenta non sono riconoscibili le piccole parti fetali

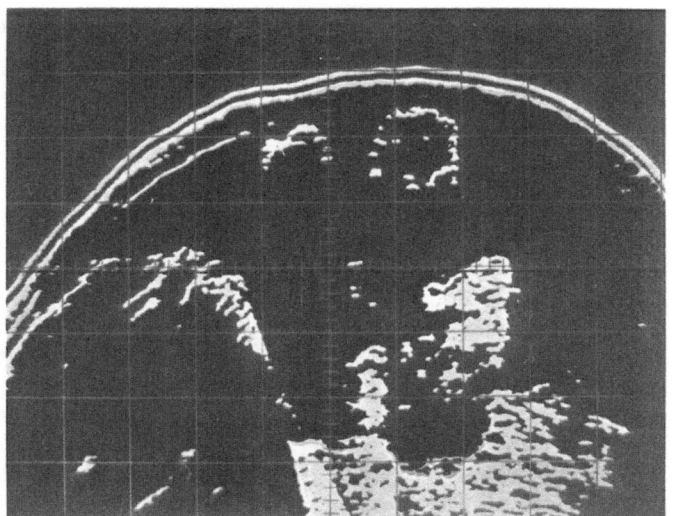

88

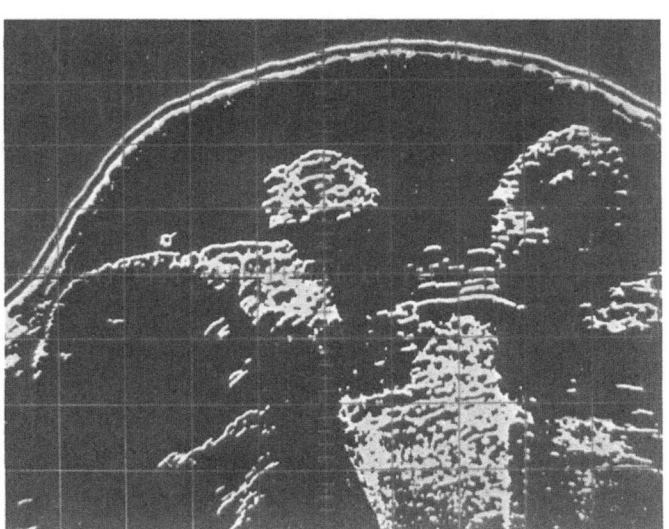

89

Intra-Uterine Death of the Fetus

Intrauteriner Fruchttod
Mort foetale intra-utérine
Muerte fetal intrauterina
Morte intrauterina del feto

Fig. 90. Intra-Uterine Death of the Fetus

Distinct deformation and double contouring of the head of the child in an amenorrhoea of 23 weeks. Scale divisions: 1 cm/section

Abb. 90. Intrauteriner Fruchttod

Deutliche Deformierung und Doppelkonturierung des kindlichen Kopfes bei einer Amenorrhoe von 23 Wochen. Skaleneinteilung pro Feld 1 cm

Fig. 90. Mort foetale intra-utérine

Nette déformation et double contour de la tête d'enfant après une aménorrhée de 23 semaines. Graduation par champ 1 cm

Fig. 90. Muerte fetal intrauterina. Embarazo de 23 semanas

Marcada deformación de la cabeza fetal. 1 división de escala = 1 cm

Fig. 90. Morte intrauterina del feto

Deformazione evidente e doppio contorno della testa fetale. Caso dopo 23 settimane di amenorrea. Graduazione della scala di 1 cm per campo

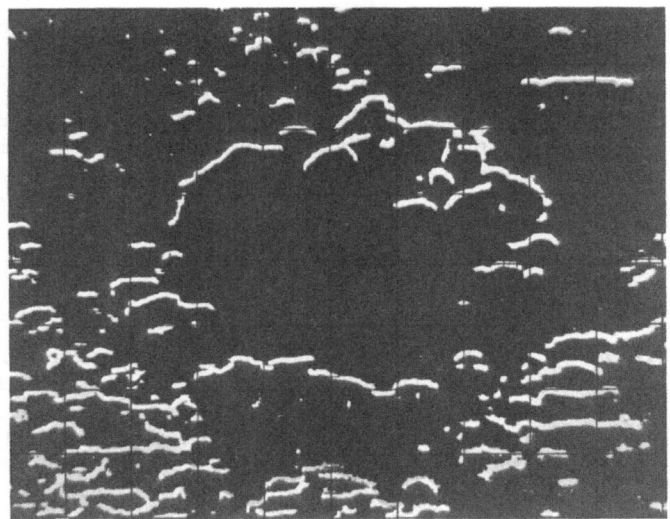

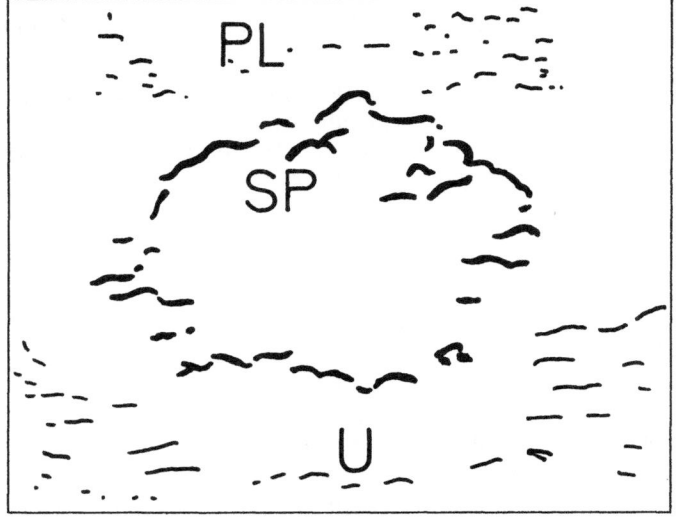

90

Fig. 91. Intra-Uterine Death of the Fetus in the 23rd Week

Cross section 2-finger widths above the symphysis. Spalding's sign and double contouring of the cranium are clearly visible. The anterior-wall placenta is above the cranium. Scale divisions are 2 cm/section

Fig. 92. Intra-Uterine Death of the Fetus in the 23rd Week

Cross section above the symphysis in the case of an intra-uterine death of the fetus in the 23nd week. Same case as Fig. 91, but with scale divisions of 1 cm/section

Abb. 91. Intrauteriner Fruchttod in der 23. Woche

Querschnitt 2 QF oberhalb der Symphyse. Spaldingsches Zeichen und Doppelkonturierung des Schädels sind deutlich zu erkennen. Oberhalb des Schädels ist die Vorderwandplacenta. Skaleneinteilung pro Feld 2 cm

Abb. 92. Intrauteriner Fruchttod in der 23. Woche

Querschnitt oberhalb der Symphyse bei einem intrauterinen Fruchttod in der 23. Woche. Gleicher Fall wie Abb. 91, jedoch mit Skaleneinteilung pro Feld 1 cm

Fig. 91. Mort foetale intra-utérine dans la 23ᵉ semaine

Coupe transversale, 2 doigts au-dessus de la symphyse. Signe de Spalding et double contour du crâne bien distincts. Le placenta ventral se trouve au-dessus du crâne. Graduation par champ 2 cm

Fig. 92. Mort foetale intra-utérine dans la 23ᵉ semaine

Coupe transversale au-dessus de la symphyse. Mort foetale intra-utérine dans la 23ᵉ semaine. Même cas que l'image 91, mais avec une graduation par champ de 1 cm

Fig. 91. Muerte fetal intrauterina — Embarazo de 23 semanas

Corte transversal 2 cm. sobre el púbis. El feto murió en la semana 23 de gestación. Se puede observar el signo de Spalding y sobre la cabeza fetal la placenta inserta en cara anterior del útero. 1 división de escala = 2 cm

Fig. 92. Muerte fetal intrauterina

Mismo caso de la figura anterior. Corte transversal suprapúbico. 1 división de escala = 1 cm

Fig. 91. Morte intrauterina del feto nella 23a settimana

Sezione trasversale 2 dita al di sopra della sinfisi pubica. Il segno di Spalding e il doppio contorno del cranio sono chiaramente visibili. Al di sopra del cranio la placenta (parete anteriore). Graduazione della scala: 2 cm per campo

Fig. 92. Morte intrauterina del feto nella 23a settimana

Sezione condotta al di sopra della sinfisi in caso di morte intrauterina del feto nella 23a settimana. Caso uguale alla Fig. 91. con graduazione di scala di 1 cm per campo

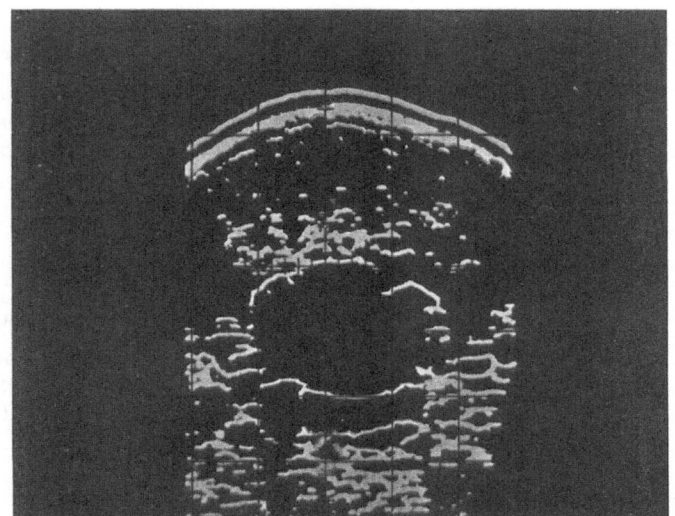

91

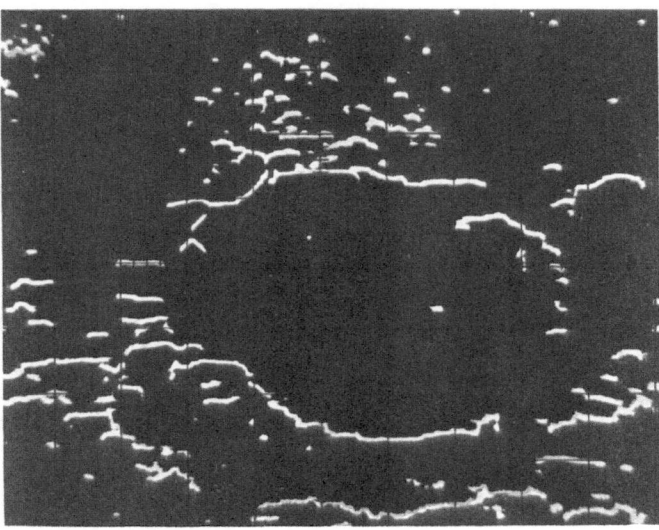

92

Fig. 93. Intra-Uterine Death of the Fetus in the 25th Week of Pregnancy

Cross section above the symphysis; same case as Fig. 90. The placenta can be seen above the cranium

Fig. 94. Intra-Uterine Death of the Fetus in the 25th Week of Pregnancy

Two-dimensional sectional diagram; same case as Fig. 91. Spalding's sign and double contouring clearly recognisable

Abb. 93. Intrauteriner Fruchttod in der 25. Woche

Querschnitt oberhalb der Symphyse. Gleicher Fall wie Abb. 90. Deformierter Schädel. Oberhalb des Schädels ist die Placenta zu erkennen

Abb. 94. Intrauteriner Fruchttod in der 25. Woche

Zweidimensionales Schnittbild. Gleicher Fall wie Abb. 91. Spaldingsches Zeichen und Doppelkontur gut zu erkennen

Fig. 93. Mort foetale intra-utérine dans la 25ᵉ semaine

Coupe transversale au-dessus de la symphyse. Même cas que l'image 90. Crâne déformé. Le placenta est visible au-dessus du crâne

Fig. 94. Mort foetale intra-utérine dans la 25ᵉ semaine

Image de coupe bidimensionnelle. Même cas que l'image 91. Signe de Spalding et double contour bien distincts

Fig. 93. Muerte fetal intrauterina — Embarazo de 25 semanas

Mismo caso de la figura 90. Corte transversal suprapúbico. Se puede observar la deformación de la cabeza fetal. Inserción de la placenta en cara anterior del útero

Fig. 94. Muerte fetal intrauterina — Embarazo de 25 semanas

Mismo caso de la figura 91. Se puede observar el signo de Spalding

Fig. 93. Morte intrauterina del feto nella 25a settimana

Sezione condotta al di sopra della sinfisi pubica. Caso eguale alla Fig. 90. Cranio deformato. Al di sopra del cranio si riconosce la placenta

Fig. 94. Morte intrauterina del feto nella 25a settimana

Quadro di sezione bidimensionale. Caso eguale alla Fig. 91. Il segno di Spalding e il doppio contorno sono chiaramente riconoscibili

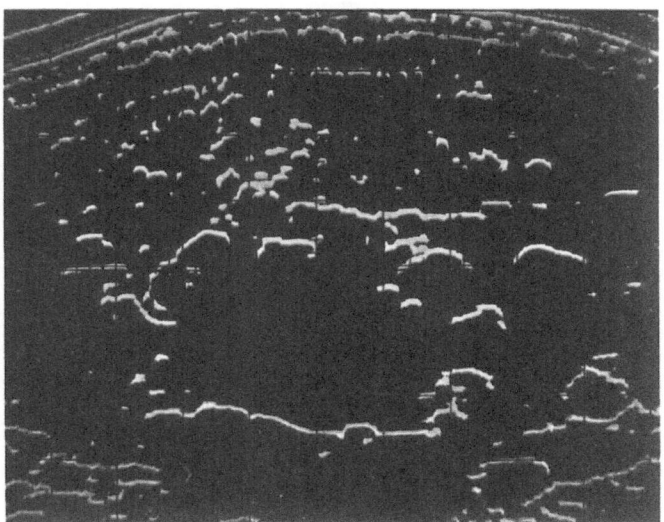

93

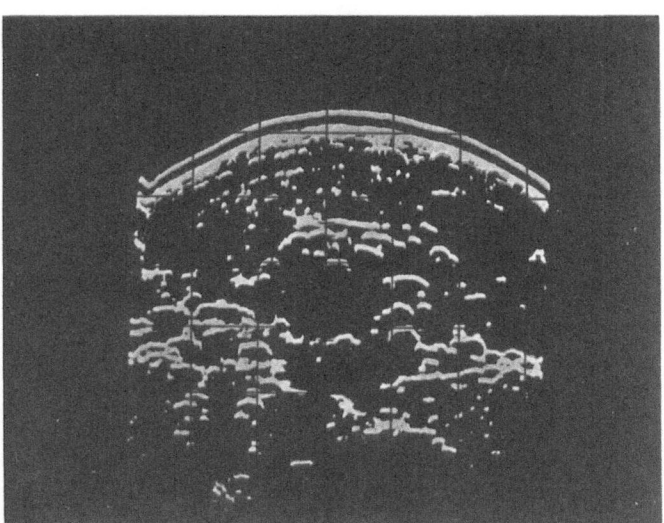

94

**Fig. 95. Intra-Uterine Death of the Fetus
in the 25th Week of Pregnancy**

Same case as Fig. 92. Cranial walls moving
closer together. Placenta clearly visible above
the cranium

Abb. 95. Intrauteriner Fruchttod in der 25. Woche

Gleicher Fall wie Abb. 92. Schädelwände rücken
näher aneinander. Placenta oberhalb des Schädels gut zu erkennen

**Fig. 95. Mort foetale intra-utérine dans la
25ᵉ semaine**

Même cas que l'image 92. Les parois du crâne
se rapprochent. Placenta bien visible au-dessus
du crâne

**Fig. 95. Muerte fetal intrauterina — Embarazo
de 25 semanas**

Mismo caso de la figura 92. Se puede observar
la deformación de la cabeza fetal, sobre la cual
se encuentra la placenta

**Fig. 95. Morte intrauterina del feto nella 25a setti-
mana**

Caso eguale alla Fig. 92. Le pareti craniali sono
accostate l'una all'altra, la placenta é riconoscibile al di sopra del cranio

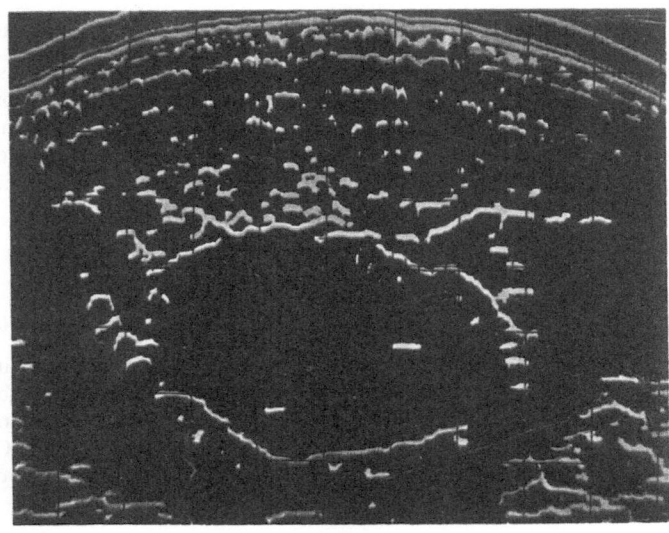

95

Abortions—Carneous Moles

Aborte — Windmole
Avortements — Faux germes
Aborto y huevo huero
Aborto — Mola ventosa

Fig. 96. Abortus Incompletus

Longitudinal section in the median line in the case of an incomplete abortion in the 10th week. The uterus can be seen underneath the overfilled bladder. The echos in the uterine cavity come from the remains of the placenta

Abb. 96. Abortus incompletus

Längsschnitt in der Medianlinie bei einem inkompletten Abort in der 10. Woche. Unterhalb der überfüllten Harnblase ist der Uterus sichtbar. Die im Cavum uteri befindlichen Echos stammen von den Placentarresten

Fig. 96. Avortement incomplet

Coupe longitudinale dans la ligne médiane. Avortement incomplet dans la 10e semaine. Sous la vessie engorgée on aperçoit l'utérus. Les échos situés dans la cavité utérine proviennent des restes placentaires

Fig. 96. Aborto incompleto

Corte longitudinal en línea media infraumbilical. Amenorrea de 10 semanas. Debajo de la vejiga llena se encuentra la matriz en cuya cavidad se pueden observar ecos provenientes de restos placentarios

Fig. 96. Aborto incompleto

Sezione longitudinale sulla linea mediana in caso di aborto incompleto nella 10a settimana di gravidanza. Al di sotto della vescica urinaria riempita al massimo é visibile l'utero. Gli echi presenti nella cavità uterina derivano da resti della placenta

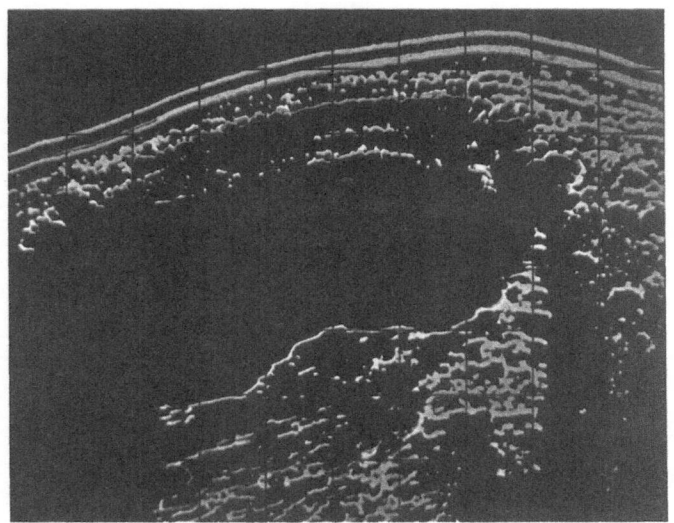

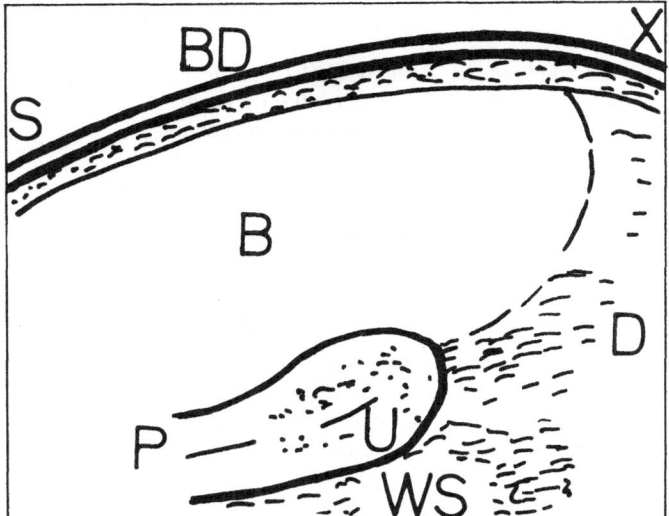

96

Fig. 97. Abortus incompletus

Cross section 2-finger widths above the symphysis, same case as Fig. 96. In the cavum uteri there are multiple echos that arise from the remains of the placenta. Scale divisions 2 cm/section

Abb. 97. Abortus incompletus

Querschnitt 2 Querfinger oberhalb der Symphyse, gleicher Fall wie Abb. 96. Im Cavum uteri befinden sich multiple Echos, die von den Placentarresten stammen. Skaleneinteilung pro Feld 2 cm

Fig. 97. Avortement incomplet

Coupe transversale, 2 doigts en-dessous de la symphyse. Même cas que l'image 96. La cavité utérine contient des échos multiples provenant des restes placentaires. Graduation par champ 2 cm

Fig. 97. Aborto incompleto

Mismo caso de la figura 96. Corte transversal 2 cm. sobre el púbis. En la cavidad uterina aparecen ecos múltiples provenientes de restos placentarios. 1 división de escala = 2 cm

Fig. 97. Aborto incompleto

Sezione trasversale 2 dita al di sopra della sinfisi. Caso uguale alla Fig. 96. Presenza di molteplici echi nella cavità uterina di derivazione placentare (resti di placenta). Graduazione della scala: 2 cm per campo

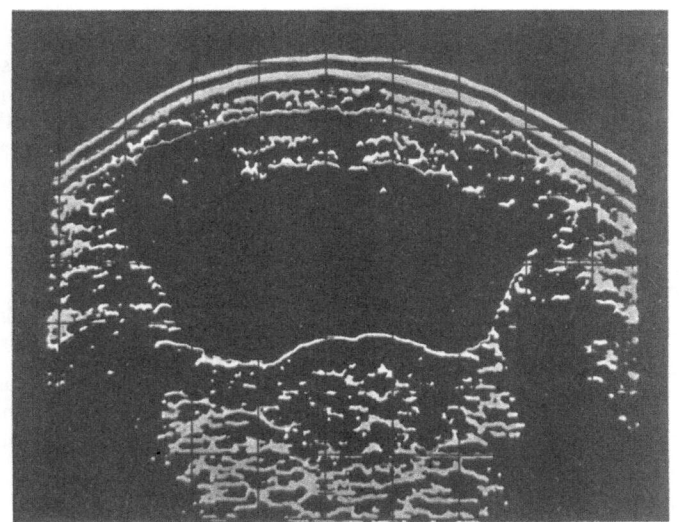

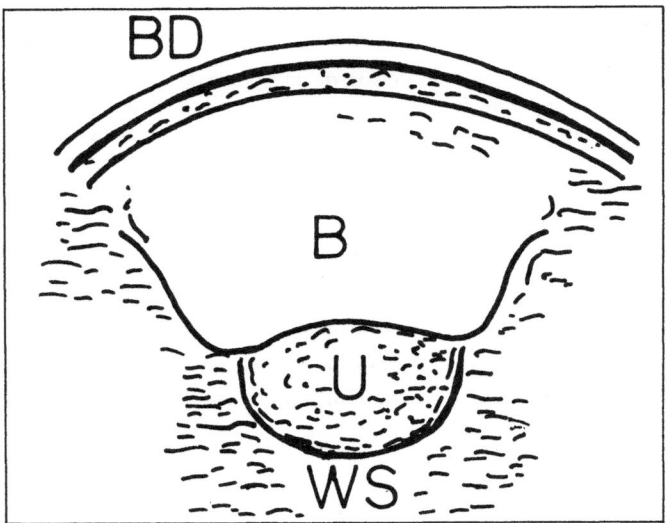

97

Fig. 98. Carneous Mole in the 10th Week

Cross section above the symphysis with full bladder. In the cavum uteri there is an empty, round embryonic sac, showing no echos and lakking the embryonic parts

Fig. 99. Carneous Mole in the 10th Week

Longitudinal section from the navel toward the symphysis, with full bladder; same case as Fig. 98. Here there is a deformed embryonic sac with trophoblast parts in the uterine cavity

Abb. 98. Windmole in der 10. Woche

Querschnitt oberhalb der Symphyse bei voller Harnblase. Im Cavum uteri befindet sich eine leere, runde, echofreie Fruchtblase mit fehlender Embryonalanlage

Abb. 99. Windmole in der 10. Woche

Längsschnitt von Nabel Richtung Symphyse, bei voller Harnblase, gleicher Fall wie Abb. 98. Hier befindet sich im Cavum ein deformierter Fruchtsack mit Trophoblastanteilen

Fig. 98. Faux germe dans la 10ᵉ semaine

Coupe transversale au-dessus de la symphyse avec vessie pleine. La cavité utérine contient une cavité amniotique vide, ronde et exempte d'échos; l'ébauche embryonnaire manque

Fig. 99. Faux germe dans la 10ᵉ semaine

Coupe longitudinale, du nombril en direction de la symphyse, avec vessie pleine. Même cas que l'image 98. Ici, la cavité contient une cavité amniotique déformée avec des éléments de trophoblastes

Fig. 98. Huevo huero — 10 semanas de amenorrea

Corte transversal suprapúbico. Paciente con vejiga llena. En la cavidad amniótuca no se observan estructuras fetales

Fig. 99. Huevo huero — 10 semanas de amenorrea

Mismo caso de la figura anterior. Corte longitudinal en línea media infraumbilical. Paciente con vejiga llena. En la cavidad amniótica se encuentran estructuras del trofoblasto

Fig. 98. Mola ventosa nella 10a settimana

Sezione al di sopra della sinfisi pubica, con vescica urinaria piena. Nella cavità uterina si trova un sacco amniotico vuoto, rotondeggiante, assolutamente privo di eco, con mancanza di embrione

Fig. 99. Mola ventosa nella 10a settimana

Sezione longitudinale dall'ombelico in direzione della sinfisi. Vescica urinaria piena. Caso uguale alla Fig. 98. Nella cavità uterina si vede un sacco amniotico deformato con elementi di trofoblasti

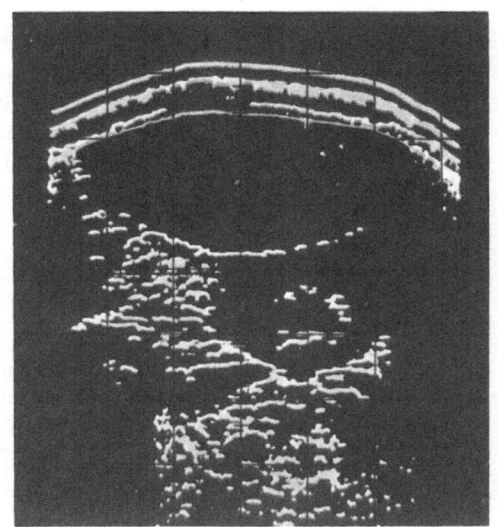
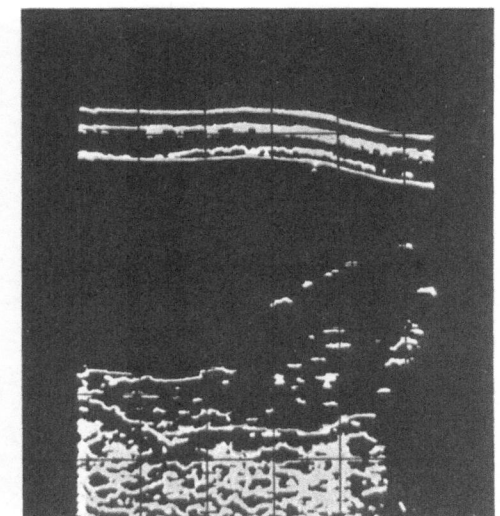

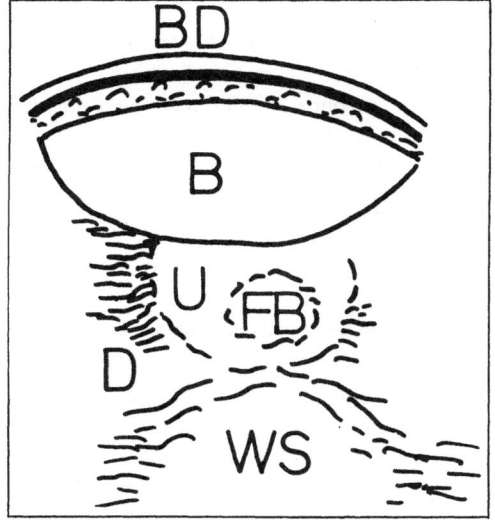
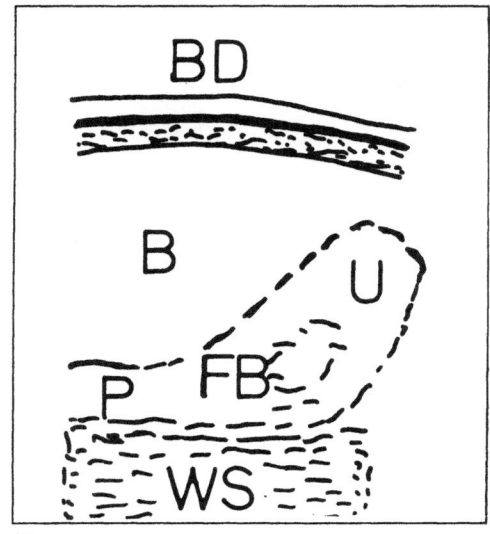

98

99

Breech Presentation

Beckenendlage
Présentation par le siège
Presentación podálica
Posizione podalica

Fig. 100. Breech Presentation in the 37th Week

Longitudinal section examination from the xiphoid toward the symphysis for diagnosis of position. The fetus' head is located in the fundus with a biparietal diameter of 8.5 cm. Scale divisions 3 cm/section. Sound frequency: 2 MHz

Abb. 100. Beckenendlage in der 37. Woche

Längsschnittuntersuchung vom Xiphoid zur Symphyse zur Lagendiagnostik. Kindlicher Kopf befindet sich im Fundus mit einem biparietalen DM von 8,5 cm. Skaleneinteilung pro Feld 3 cm. Schallfrequenz 2 MHZ

Fig. 100. Présentation par le siège dans la 37ᵉ semaine

Examen en coupe longitudinale, du xiphoïde à la symphyse, pour le diagnostic de la position. La tête d'enfant se trouve dans le fond de l'utérus, avec un diamètre bipariétal de 8,5 cm. Graduation par champ 3 cm. Fréquence de son 2 MHz

Fig. 100. Presentación podálica. Embarazo de 37 semanas

Corte longitudinal desde el xifoides hasta al púbis. El polo cefálico se encuentra en el fondo uterino y tiene un diámetro biparietal de 8,5 cm. 1 división de escala = 3 cm. Frecuencia del ultrasonido = 2 MHz

Fig. 100. Presentazione podalica nella 37a settimana

Sezione longitudinale dal processo xifoide alla sinfisi pubica. La testa del bambino si trova nel fondo dell'utero, il diametro biparietale é di 8,5 cm. Graduazione della scala 3 cm per campo. Frequenza: 2 MHZ

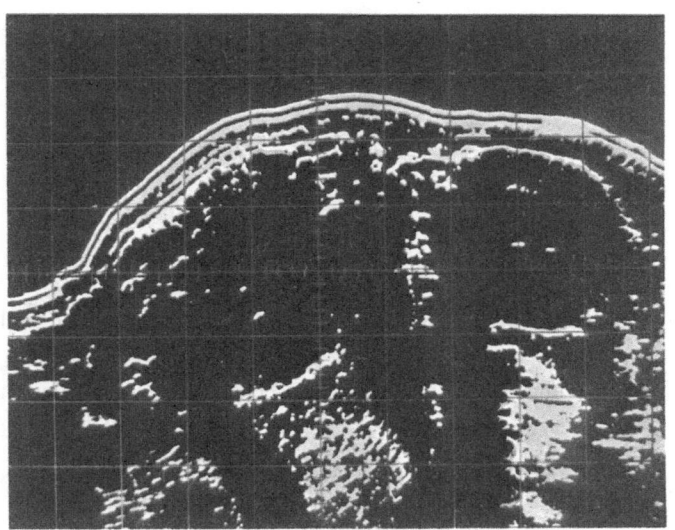

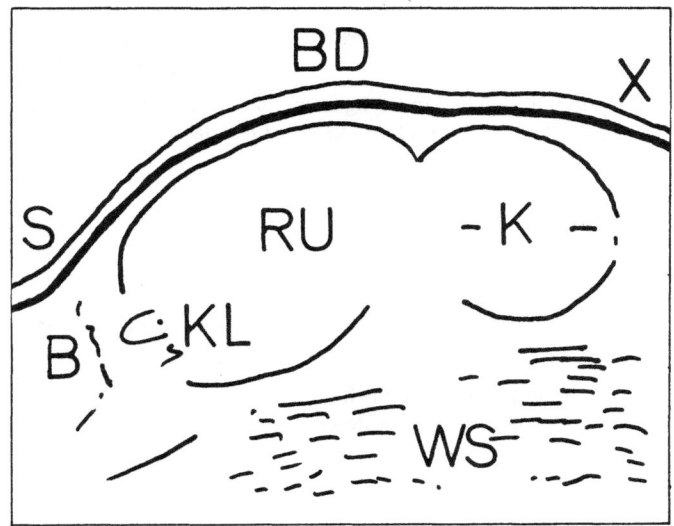

100

Fig. 101. Breech Presentation in the 38th Week

Longitudinal section in the median line; head located in the fundus. Scale divisions: 3 cm/section

Fig. 102. Breech Presentation in the 38th Week

Supraumbilical cross section with a scale division of 2 cm/section. Here the head is located in the fundus

Abb. 101. Beckenendlage in der 38. Woche

Längsschnitt in der Medianlinie, Kopf befindet sich im Fundus. Skaleneinteilung pro Feld 3 cm

Abb. 102. Beckenendlage in der 38.Woche

Supraumbilicaler Querschnitt bei einer Skaleneinteilung von 2 cm pro Feld. Hier befindet sich der Kopf im Fundus

Fig. 101. Présentation par le siège dans la 38ᵉ semaine

Coupe longitudinale dans la ligne médiane. La tête se trouve dans le fond de l'utérus. Graduation par champ 3 cm

Fig. 102. Présentation par le siège dans la 38ᵉ semaine

Coupe transversale supra-ombilicale. Graduation par champ 2 cm. La tête se trouve ici dans le fond de l'utérus

Fig. 101. Presentación podálica — Embarazo de 38 semanas

Corte longitudinal en línea media. Polo cefálico en fondo uterino. 1 división de escala = 3 cm

Fig. 102. Presentación podálica — Embarazo de 38 semans

Corte transversal supraumbilical. Polo cefálico en fondo uterino. 1 división de escala = 2 cm

Fig. 101. Presentazione podalica nella 38a settimana

Sezione longitudinale sulla linea mediana, la testa si trova sul fondo dell'utero, graduazione di scala 3 cm

Fig. 102. Presentazione podalica nella 38a settimana

Sezione sopraombelicale, con graduazione di scala di 2 cm per campo. Qui la testa si trova nel fondo dell'utero

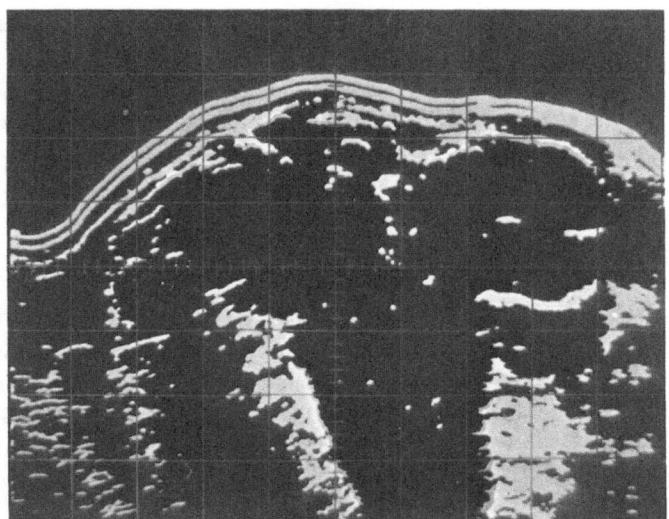

101

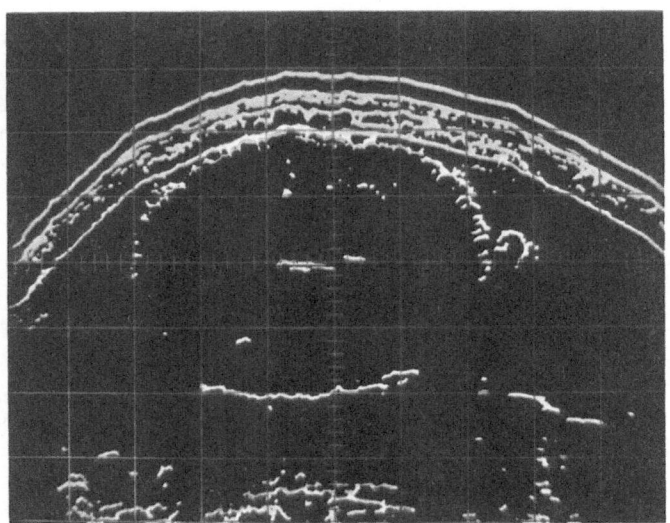

102

Fig. 103. Position of Cranium in the 38th Week

Longitudinal section in the median line; head located above the symphysis. Placenta located on the anterior wall. Scale divisions: 3 cm/section

Fig. 104. Position of Cranium in the 38th Week

Cross section above the symphysis. Whole circumference of head with central echo clearly visible. Scale divisions 2 cm/section

Abb. 103. Schädellage in der 38. Woche

Längsschnitt in der Medianlinie, Kopf befindet sich oberhalb der Symphyse. Placenta sitzt an der Vorderwand. Skaleneinteilung pro Feld 3 cm

Abb. 104. Schädellage in der 38. Woche

Querschnitt oberhalb der Symphyse. Gesamter Kopfumfang mit Mittelecho gut sichtbar. Skaleneinteilung pro Feld 2 cm

Fig. 103. Position du crâne dans la 38ᵉ semaine

Coupe longitudinale dans la ligne médiane. La tête se trouve au-dessus de la symphyse. Le placenta se trouve à la paroi ventrale. Graduation par champ 3 cm

Fig. 104. Position du crâne dans la 38ᵉ semaine

Coupe transversale au-dessus de la symphyse. La tête avec écho médian est bien visible dans toute son étendue. Graduation par champ 2 cm

Fig. 103. Presentación cefálica — Embarazo de 38 semanas

Corte longitudinal en línea media. El polo cefálico se encuentra cerca del púbis. Placenta inserta en cara anterior del útero. 1 división de escala = 3 cm

Fig. 104. Presentación cefálica — Embarazo de 38 semanas

Corte transversal suprapúbico. Cabeza fetal es visible con eco medio. 1 división de escala = 2 cm

Fig. 103. Posizione cefalica nella 38a settimana

Sezione longitudinale sulla linea mediana, la testa si trova al di sopra della sinfisi. La placenta é situata sulla parete anteriore. Graduazione di scala 3 cm

Fig. 104. Presentazione cefalica nella 38a settimana

Sezione condotta al di sopra della sinfisi. Diametro cefalico in toto visibile con l'eco medio. Graduazione di scala: 2 cm per campo

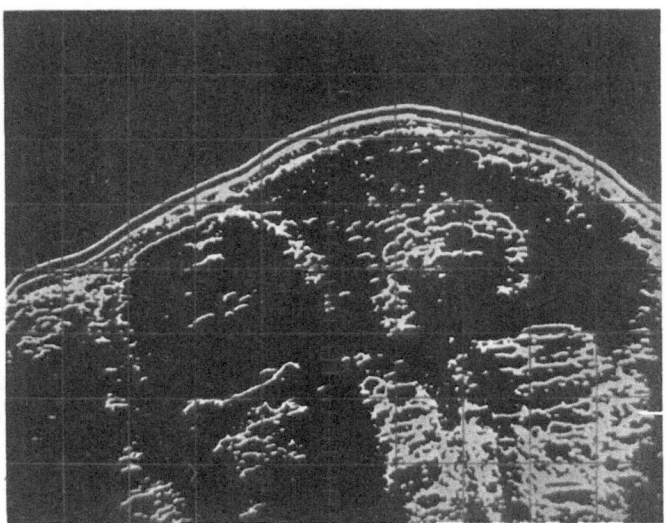

103

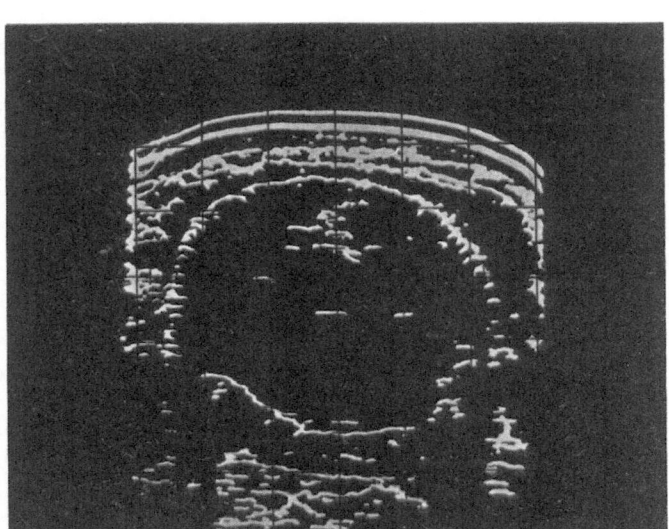

104

Fig. 105. Breech Presentation with Bicornuate Uterus

Cross section at level of fundus with breech presentation and uterus bicornis in the 40th week. Head is in the fundus, namely in the left-hand horn. Beside the head, the septum between the left- and right-hand horns is visible. Scale divisions 2 cm/section. The radiograph shows the findings 3 months post partum

Abb. 105. Beckenendlage bei Uterus bicornis

Querschnitt in Fundushöhe bei Beckenendlage und Uterus bicornis in der 40. Woche. Kopf befindet sich im Fundus, und zwar im linken Horn. Neben dem Kopf ist das Septum zwischen linkem und rechtem Horn sichtbar. Skaleneinteilung pro Feld 2 cm. Die Röntgenaufnahme zeigt den Befund 3 Monate post partum

Fig. 105. Présentation par le siège avec uterus bicornis

Coupe transversale à hauteur du fond de l'utérus dans la 40e semaine. Présentation par le siège avec uterus bicornis. La tête se trouve dans le fond de l'utérus et notamment dans la corne de gauche. A côté de la tête on aperçoit la cloison séparant les cornes de gauche et de droite. Graduation par champ 2 cm. La radiographie montre la situation, 3 mois après l'accouchement

Fig. 105. Presentación podálica con útero bicornio

Embarazo de 40 semanas. Corte transversal a nivel del fondo uterino. El polo cefálico se encuentra en el fondo uterino al lado del tabique que separa al cuerno derecho del izquierdo. La histerosalpingografía fué hecha 3 meses postparto. 1 división de escala = 2 cm

Fig. 105. Presentazione podalica in caso di utero bicorne

Sezione condotta al livello del fondo dell'utero. La testa si trova sul fondo e cioé nel corno sinistro Accanto alla testa é visibile il setto separante i due corni. Graduazione di scala 2 cm. per campo. La radiografia mostra come si presenta la situazione 3 mesi dopo il parto

Fig. 106. Breech Presentation with Bicornuate Uterus

Cross section at level of fundus, same case as Fig. 105. Here the scale divisions are 3 cm/section. The partition between the left- and right-hand horns is clearly visible

Abb. 106. Beckenendlage bei Uterus bicornis

Querschnitt in Fundushöhe. Gleicher Fall wie Abb. 105. Hier beträgt Skaleneinteilung pro Feld 3 cm. Trennwand zwischen linkem und rechtem Horn gut zu erkennen

Fig. 106. Présentation par le siège avec uterus bicornis

Coupe transversale à hauteur du fond de l'utérus. Même cas que l'image 105. La graduation par champ mesure ici 3 cm. La cloison de séparation entre les cornes de gauche et de droite est bien distincte

Fig. 106. Presentación podálica con útero bicornio

Mismo caso de la figura anterior. Corte transversal a nivel de fondo uterino. Se puede observar el tabique divisorio de los dos cuernos. 1 división de escala = 3 cm

Fig. 106. Presentazione podalica in caso di utero bicorne

Sezione condotta a livello del fondo. Caso uguale alla Fig. 105. La graduazione di scala é di 3 cm. per campo. Il setto separante i due corni, sinistro e destro, é qui ben visibile

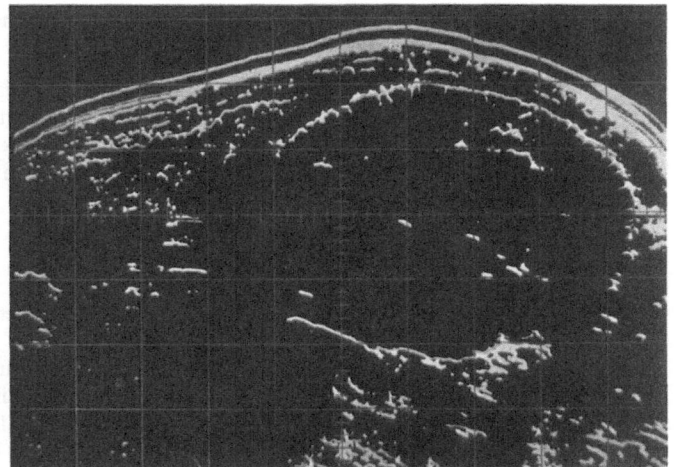

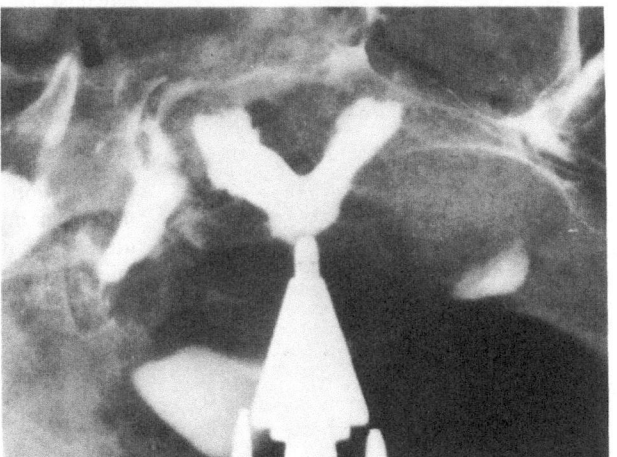

105

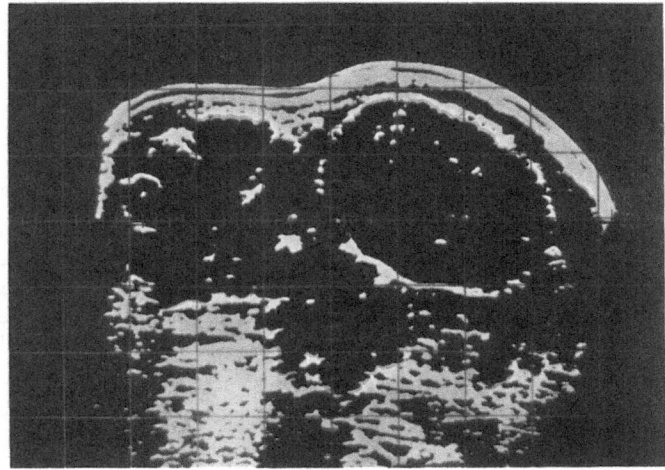

106

Malformations

Mißbildungen
Malformations
Malformaciones
Malformazioni

Fig. 107. Anencephalus in the 36th Week of Pregnancy

Presentation in logitudinal section. The greatly malformed skull is located in the Fundus uteri. The typical skull configuration is absent. Scale division: 3 cm. Sound frequency: 2.5 MHz

Abb. 107. Anencephalus in der 36. Woche

Darstellung im medianen Längsschnitt. Der stark mißgebildete Schädel befindet sich am Fundus uteri. Es fehlt die typische Schädelkonfiguration, die bei intakter Schwangerschaft zu sehen ist. Die Skaleneinteilung pro Feld beträgt 3 cm. Schallfrequenz $2^1/_2$ MHZ

Fig. 107. Anencéphale dans la 36ᵉ semaine de grossesse

Présentation en coupe longitudinale. Le crâne fortement malformé est situé dans le Fundus uteri. La configuration typique du crâne manque. Division de l'échelle: 3 cm. Fréquence du son: 2,5 MHz

Fig. 107. Anencéfalo. Embarazo de 36 semanas

Corte longitudinal. Podálica. El cráneo fetal presenta malformaciones muy marcadas y se encuentra en el fondo uterino. Además falta la configuración cefálica típica. 1 división de escala = 3 cm. Frecuencia del ultrasonido = 2,5 MHz

Fig. 107. Anencefalo nella 36a settimana

Sezione longitudinale sulla linea mediana. Il cranio malformato si trova sul fondo dell'utero. Manca la configurazione tipica del cranio, come si osserva nella gravidanza normale. Graduazione della scala: 3 cm per campo. Frequenza 2,5 MHZ

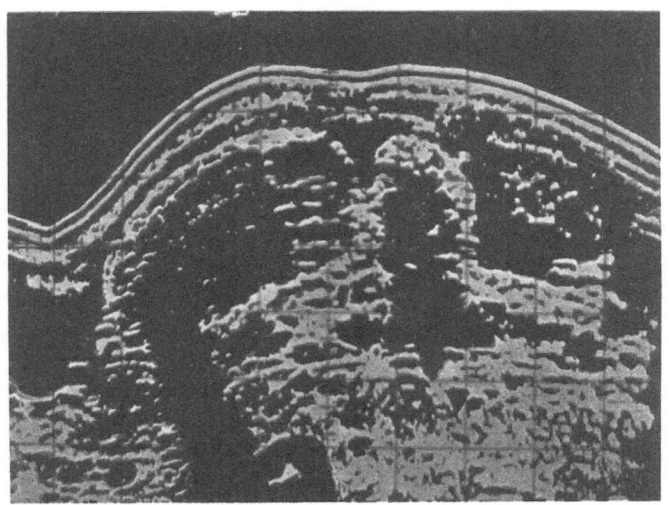

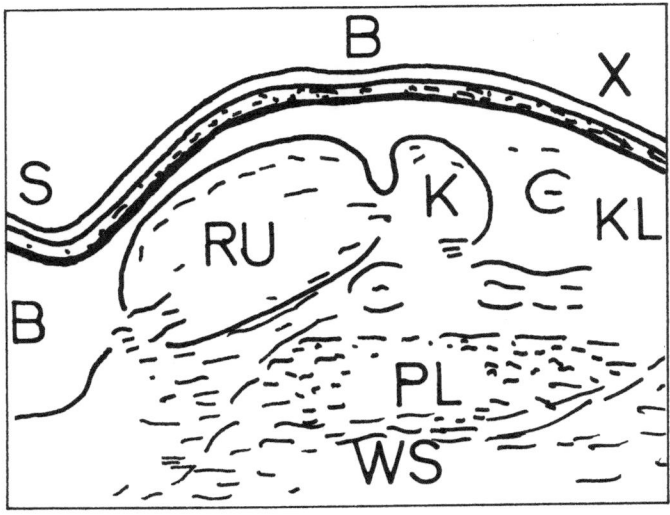

107

Measuring the True Conjugate

Messung der Conjugata vera
Mesurage du diamètre antéro-postérieur
Medición del verdadero conjugado
Misurazione della coniugata vera

Fig. 108. Measuring the True Conjugate by B-scan

Longitudinal section in the median line with a uterus 4 weeks post partum and a full bladder. The upper arrow shows the posterior wall of the symphysis, the lower arrow the promontorium. Scale divisions: 2 cm per section; true conjugate: 10.7 cm (also 10.7 cm when measured radiographically)

Abb. 108. Messung der Conjugata vera mit B-Bild

Längsschnitt in der Medianlinie bei einem Uterus 4 Wochen post partum und mit voller Blase. Der obere Pfeil zeigt die hintere Wand der Symphyse, der untere Pfeil das Promontorium. Skaleneinteilung pro Feld 2 cm, Conjugata vera 10,7 cm (röntgenologisch gemessen ebenfalls 10,7 cm)

Fig. 108. Mesurage du diamètre antéro-postérieur par image B

Coupe longitudinale dans la ligne médiane d'un utérus, 4 semaines post-partum et avec vessie pleine. La flèche supérieure indique la paroi postérieure de la symphyse, la flèche inférieure le promontoire. Graduation par champ 2 cm. Diamètre antéro-postérieur 10,7 cm (le mesurage radiologique donne également 10,7 cm)

Fig. 108. Medición del conjugado verdadero — Imagen B

4 semanas post parto. Corte longitudinal en línea media. Vejiga llena. La flecha superior marca la superficie posterior del pubis, la flecha inferior, el promontorio. Conjugado verdadero: 10,7 cm. (Con ultrasonido y rayos X). 1 división de escala = 2 cm

Fig. 108. Misurazione della coniugata vera ottenuta mediante l'immagine b

Sezione longitudinale sulla linea mediana. Utero 4 settimane dopo il parto, vescica urinaria piena. La freccia superiore indica la parete posteriore della sinfisi pubica, quella inferiore indica il promontorio. Graduazione della scala 2 cm per campo, coniugata vera 10,7 cm (Lunghezza perfettamente eguale a quella ottenuta per via radiologica)

Fig. 109. Measuring the True Conjugate by A-Diagram

Same case as Fig. 108; but measured by A-diagram. Here the sound head is applied to the symphysis pointing toward the promontorium. The first large echo of high amplitude corresponds to the posterior wall of the symphysis. The second echo of high amplitude corresponds to the promontorium. Here the conjugata vera is 10.7 cm, scale divisions 2 cm/section

Abb. 109. Messung der Conjugata vera mit A-Bild

Gleicher Fall wie Abb. 108, jedoch Messung mit A-Bild. Hier wird der Schallkopf von der Symphyse aus in Richtung Promontorium angesetzt. Das erste große Echo mit hoher Amplitude entspricht der Symphysenhinterwand. Das zweite Echo mit hoher Amplitude entspricht dem Promontorium. Conjugata vera beträgt hier 10,7 cm, Skaleneinteilung pro Feld 2 cm

Fig. 109. Mesurage du diamètre antéro-postérieur par image A

Même cas que l'image 108, mais mesuré à l'aide de l'image A. Ici, la tête sonore est appliquée sur la symphyse et orientée vers le promontoire. Le premier grand écho à grande amplitude correspond à la paroi postérieure de la symphyse. Le second écho à haute amplitude correspond au promontoire. Le diamètre antéro-postérieur mesure ici 10,7 cm. Graduation par champ 2 cm

Fig. 109. Medición del conjugado verdadero. Imagen A

Mismo caso de la figura anterior. El transductor se apoya sobre el pubis en dirección hacia el promontorio. El primer eco de gran amplitud representa la superficie posterior del pubis. El segundo eco de gran amplitud representa al promontorio. Conjugado verdadero: 10,7 cm. 1 división de escala = 2 cm

Fig. 109. Misurazione della coniugata vera con l'immagine A

Caso uguale alla Fig. 108, solo la misurazione é ottenuta mediante l'immagine A. Qui la testina esploratrice viene manovrata partendo dalla sinfisi in direzione del promontorio. Il primo grande eco caratterizzato da una grande amplitudine corrisponde alla parete interna della sinfisi. Il secondo eco, di eguale grande amplitudine, corrisponde al promontorio. La coniugata vera é di 10,7 cm. Graduazione della scala di 2 cm per campo

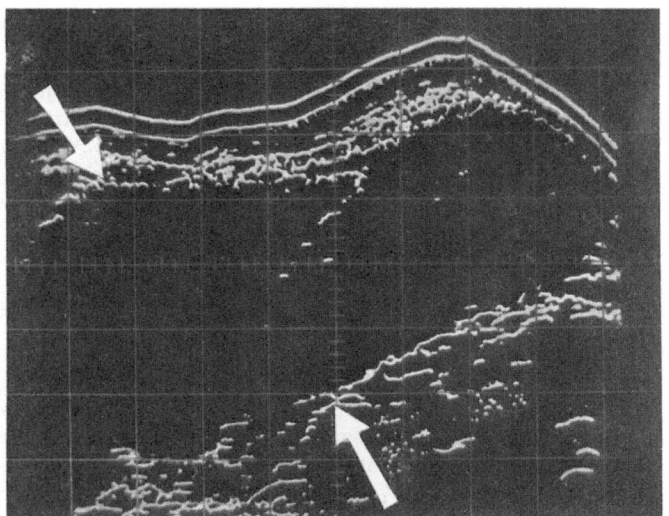

108

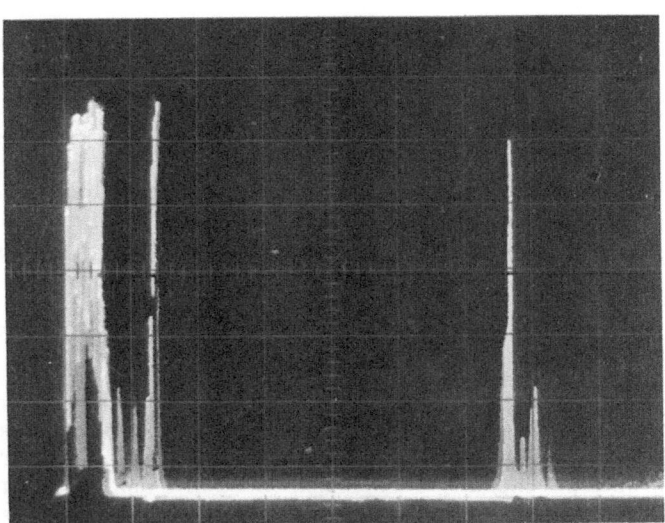

109

Fig. 110. Measuring the True Conjugate by A-scan

Sound head acting from the symphysis toward the promontorium with full bladder. The distance between the two echos corresponds to the distance from the posterior wall of the symphysis to the promontorium. True conjugate: 12 cm. Radiographic measurement of the pelvis gave a true conjugate of 11.9 cm

Fig. 111. Measuring the True Conjugate by B-scan

Longitudinal section in the median line in a pregnancy in the 37th week. The upper arrow denotes the rear wall of the symphysis, the lower arrow the promontorium. The distance corresponds to a true conjugate of 12 cm. Scale divisions: 3 cm, section

Abb. 110. Messung der Conjugata vera mit A-Bild

Schallkopf von der Symphyse aus in Richtung Promontorium mit voller Harnblase. Die Entfernung der beiden Echos entspricht der Distanz Symphysenhinterwand zu Promontorium. Conjugata vera: 12 cm. Die röntgenologische Beckenmessung ergab eine Conjugata vera von 11,9 cm

Abb. 111. Messung der Conjugata vera mit B-Bild

Längsschnitt in der Medianlinie bei einer Schwangerschaft in der 37. Woche. Der obere Pfeil bezeichnet die Symphysenhinterwand, der untere Pfeil das Promontorium. Die Entfernung entspricht Conjugata vera von 12 cm. Skaleneinteilung pro Feld 3 cm

Fig. 110. Mesurage du diamètre antéro-postérieur par image A

Tête sonore appliquée sur la symphyse et orientée vers le promontoire. Vessie pleine. L'espacement des deux échos correspond à la distance paroi postérieure de la symphyse / promontoire. Diamètre antéro-postérieur: 12 cm. La pelvimétrie radiologique indiquait un diamètre antéropostérieur de 11,9 cm

Fig. 111. Mesurage du diamètre antéro-postérieur par image B

Coupe longitudinale dans la ligne médiane dans la 37e semaine d'une grossesse. La flèche supérieure indique la paroi postérieure de la symphyse, la flèche inférieure le promontoire. La distance correspond à un diamètre antéropostérieur de 12 cm. Graduation par champ 3 cm

Fig. 110. Medición del conjugado verdadero. Imagen A

Transductor sobre el pubis en dirección hacia el promontorio. Vejiga llena. La distancia de ambos ecos corresponde a la distancia entre superficie posterior del pubis y promontorio. Conjugado verdadero: 12,0 cm. con ltrasonido, 11,9 cm con rayos X

Fig. 111. Medición del conjugado verdadero. Imagen B

Corte longitudinal en línea media. Embarazo de 37 semanas de gestación. La flecha superior señala la superficie posterior del pubis, la flecha inferior marca el promontorio. Conjugado verdadero: 12,0 cm. 1 división de escala = 3 cm

Fig. 110. Misurazione della coniugata vera mediante l'immagine A

Testina esploratrice dalla sinfisi in direzione del promontorio, vescica urinaria riempita al massimo. La distanza che separa i due echi, corrisponde alla distanza tra la parete interna della sinfisi e il promontorio. Coniugata vera: 12 cm. Con la misurazione radiografica si è ottenuta una coniugata vera di 11,9 cm

Fig. 111. Misurazione della coniugata vera mediante l'immagine B.

Sezione longitudinale sulla linea mediana in caso di gravidanza nella 37ma settimana. La freccia superiore indica la parete interna della sinfisi, la freccia inferiore il promontorio. La distanza tra i due punti corrisponde ad una coniugata vera di 12 cm. Graduazione di scala: 3 cm per campo

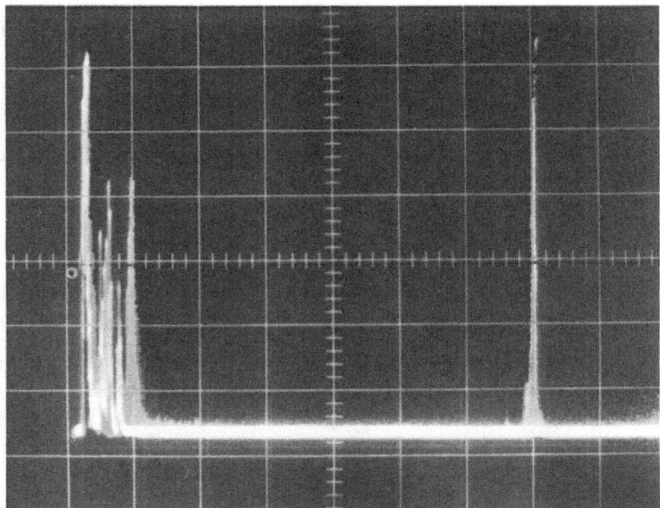

110

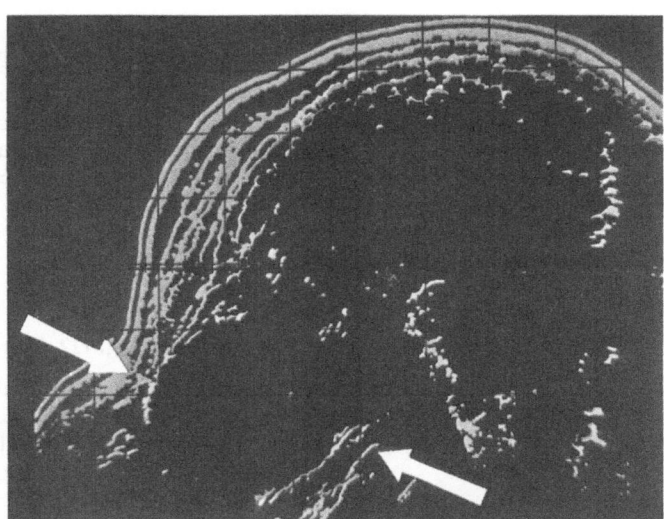

111

Involution of the Uterus during the Puerperium

Involution des Uterus im Wochenbett
Involution de l'utérus en couches
Involución uterina en el puerperio
Involuzione dell'utero nel puerperio

Fig. 112. Uterus Post Partum

Longitudinal section in the median line in the case of a uterus 2 days post partum. Dash-like echos in the uterus correspond to the cavum uteri. Full bladder beyond the uterus

Abb. 112. Uterus post partum

Längsschnitt in der Medianlinie bei einem Uterus 2 Tage post partum. Strichförmige Echos im Uterus entsprechen dem Cavum. Caudal vom Uterus volle Harnblase

Fig. 112. Utérus post-partum

Coupe longitudinale, dans la ligne médiane, d'un utérus 2 jours post-partum. Echos en forme de traits dans l'utérus, correspondant à la cavité. En direction caudale de l'utérus: la vessie pleine

Fig. 112. Utero post parto

Corte longitudinal en línea media. Parto hace 2 dias. Los ecos en línea corresponden a la cavidad uterina. En dirección caudal se encuentra la vejiga llena

Fig. 112. Utero dopo il parto

Sezione longitudinale sulla linea mediana in utero due giorni dopo il parto. Eco di tipo lineare nell'utero corrispondente alla cavità uterina. Caudalmente all'utero si vede la vescica urinaria piena

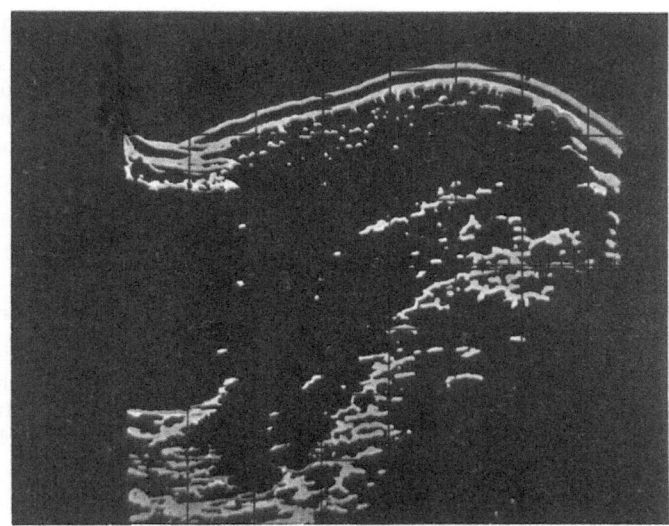

112

Fig. 113. Uterus Post Partum

Cross section above the symphysis with a uterus 2 days post partum. Same case as Fig. 112. Scale divisions: 2 cm/section

Fig. 114. Uterus Post Partum

Longitudinal section with a uterus on the 4th day post partum. Same case as Fig. 112. The progress of involution is clearly recognisable. Full bladder beyond the uterus

Abb. 113. Uterus post partum

Querschnitt oberhalb der Symphyse bei einem Uterus 2 Tage post partum. Gleicher Fall wie Abb. 112. Skaleneinteilung pro Feld 2 cm

Abb. 114. Uterus post partum

Längsschnitt bei einem Uterus am 4. Tag post partum. Gleicher Fall wie Abb. 112. Der Involutionsfortschritt ist gut zu erkennen. Caudal vom Uterus volle Harnblase

Fig. 113. Utérus post-partum

Coupe transversale au-dessus de la symphyse d'un utérus 2 jours post-partum. Même cas que l'image 112. Graduation par champ 2 cm

Fig. 114. Utérus post-partum

Coupe longitudinale d'un utérus au 4e jour post-partum. Même cas que l'image 112. La progression de l'involution est bien perceptible. En direction caudale de l'utérus: la vessie pleine

Fig. 113. Utero post parto

Mismo caso de la figura anterior. Parto hace 2 dias. Corte transversal suprapúbico. 1 división de escala = 2 cm

Fig. 114. Utero post parto

Mismo caso de la figura 112. Parto hace 4 dias. Corte longitudinal en línea media. Se puede observar la involución uterina. En dirección caudal se encuentra la vejiga

Fig. 113. Utero dopo il parto

Sezione condotta al di sopra della sinfisi due giorni dopo il parto. Esempio uguale alla Fig. 112. Graduazione della scala: 2 cm per campo

Fig. 114. Utero dopo il parto

Sezione longitudinale quattro giorni dopo il parto. Caso uguale alla Fig. 112. L'involuzione subita dall'utero é chiaramente riconoscibile, caudalmente all'utero é visibile la vescica urinaria

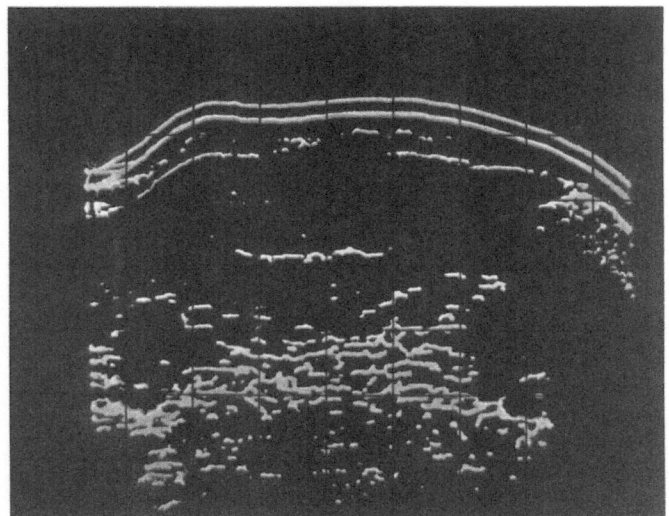

113

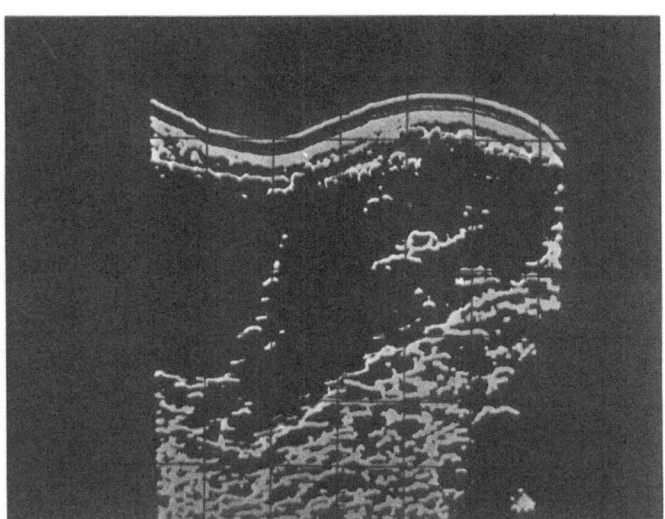

114

Fig. 115. Uterus Post Partum

Cross section above the symphysis on the 4th
day post partum; same case as Fig. 113. Scale
divisions: 2 cm/section

Abb. 115. Uterus post partum

Suprasymphysärer Querschnitt am 4. Tag post
partum. Gleicher Fall wie Abb. 113. Skaleneinteilung pro Feld 2 cm

Fig. 115. Utérus post-partum

Coupe transversale suprasymphysaire au 4ᵉ jour
post-partum. Même cas que l'image 113. Graduation par champ 2 cm

Fig. 115. Utero post parto

Mismo caso de la figura 113. Parto hace 4 dias.
Corte transversal suprapúbico. 1 división de escala = 2 cm

Fig. 115. Utero dopo il parto

Sezione soprasinfisaria quattro giorni dopo il
parto. Caso uguale alla Fig. 113. Graduazione
della scala: 2 cm per campo

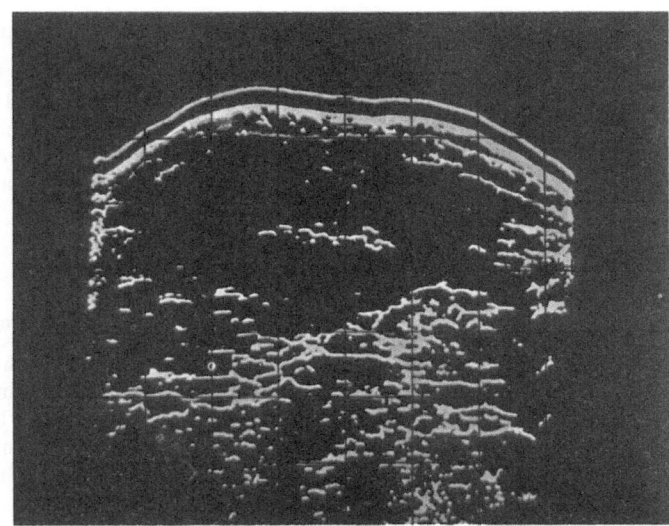

115

Ultrasonic Diagnosis in Gynecology

Ultraschalldiagnostik in der Gynäkologie
Diagnostic à ultrasons en gynécologie
Diagnóstico ultrasónico en ginecología
L'ecografia al servizio della ginecologia

Fig. 116. Myoma with Necrosis

Ultrasonic echogram in longitudinal section from the navel toward the symphysis with a large uterine myoma. The echos in the region of the lower section of the body correspond to the necrosis. The bladder is below

Abb. 116. Myom mit Nekrose

Ultraschallechogramm im Längsschnitt vom Nabel Richtung Symphyse bei großem Uterus myomatosus. Die Echos im Bereich des unteren Korpusabschnittes entsprechen der Nekrose. Caudal liegt die Harnblase

Fig. 116. Myome avec nécrose

Echogramme à ultrasons en coupe longitudinale du nombril vers la symphyse. Grand utérus myomateux. Les échos dans la zone de la section inférieure du corps correspondent à la nécrose. La vessie se trouve en direction caudale

Fig. 116. Mioma con necrosis

Corte longitudinal en línea media infraumbilical. Se puede observar el útero miomatose, los ecos en la parte inferior del útero corresponden a zonas de necrosis. En dirección caudal se encuentra la vejiga

Fig. 116. Mioma uterino con necrosi

Ecogramma in sezione longitudinale, in partenza dall'ombelico e in direzione della sinfisi in caso di grosso utero miomatoso. Gli echi in prossimità della parte inferiore della sezione del corpo uterino corrispondono alla parte necrotica. Caudalmente la vescica urinaria

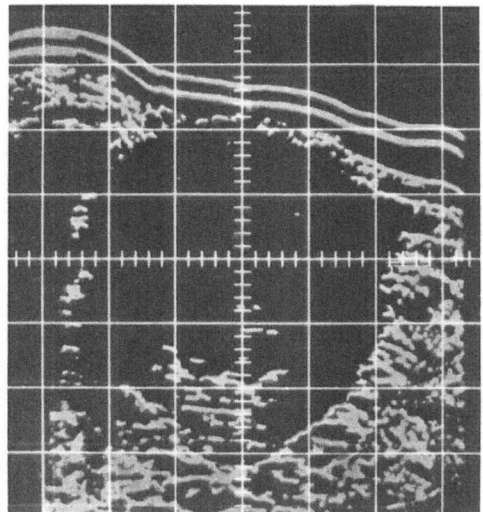

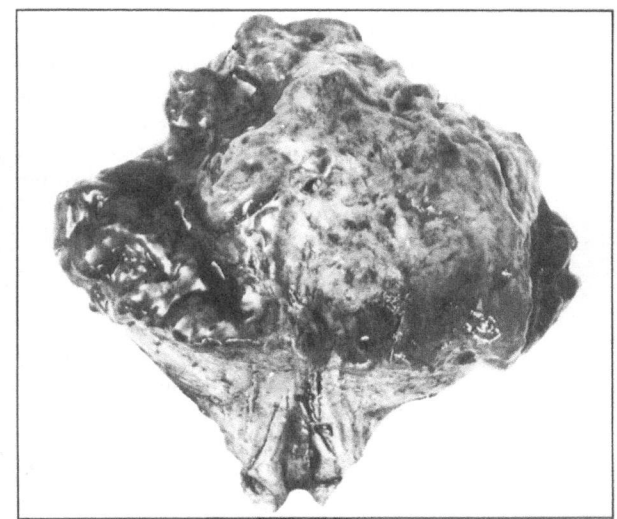

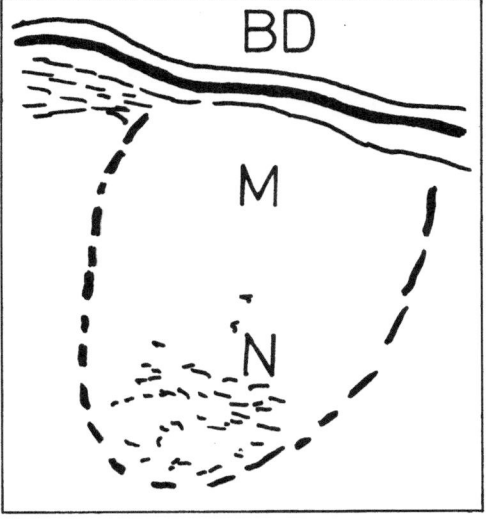

116

Fig. 117. Uterine myoma

Longitudinal section in the median line with large uterine myoma with bowing forward of the posterior wall. The echos which are to be seen in the lower third of the myoma correspond to the boundaries of the large nodules. Scale division: 2 cm/section

Abb. 117. Uterus myomatosus

Längsschnitt in der Medianlinie bei großem Uterus myomatosus mit Vorwölbung von der Hinterwand nach vorne. Die Echos, die im caudalen Drittel des Myoms zu sehen sind, entsprechen der Begrenzung des großen Knotens. Skaleneinteilung pro Feld 2 cm

Fig. 117. Utérus myomateux

Coupe longitudinale dans la ligne médiane. Grand utérus myomateux avec bombement de la paroi postérieure vers l'avant. Les échos, visibles dans le tiers caudal du myome, correspondent à la délimitation du grand noeud. Graduation par champ 2 cm

Fig. 117. Utero miomatoso

Corte longitudinal en línea media infraumbilical. En el útero miomatoso se puede observar la deformación de la pared posterior. Los ecos del tercio caudal del mioma corresponden al nódulo mayor. 1 división de escala = 2 cm

Fig. 117. Mioma uterino

Sezione longitudinale sulla linea mediana in caso di grosso utero miomatoso, con incurvatura in avanti della parete posteriore. Gli echi che si vedono nel terzo caudale corrispondono ai limiti dati dai grossi noduli miomatosi. Graduazione di scala: 2 cm per campo

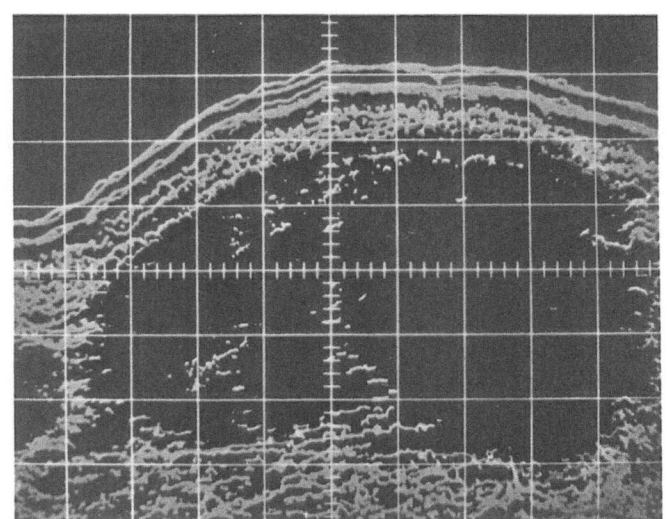

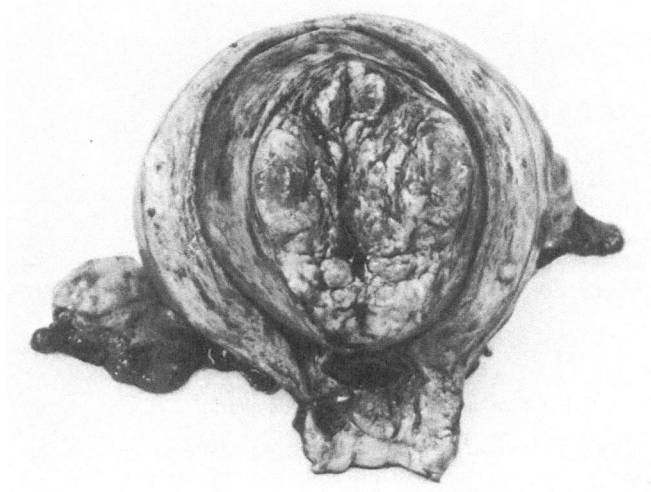

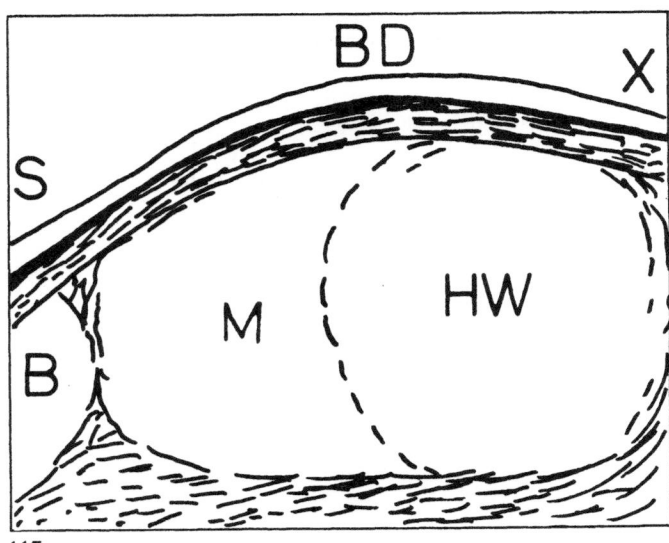

Fig. 118. Uterine Myoma with Ovarian Tumor

This is a case of a cystic, multilocular ovarian tumor, which has grown closely together with the posterior wall of the uterus. The uterus itself is coarsely nodular with large. Subserosal nodules, filling the pouch of Douglas

Abb. 118. Uterus myomatosus mit Ovarialtumor

Es handelt sich um einen cystischen, mehrkammerigen Ovarialtumor, der mit der Uterushinterwand eng verwachsen ist. Der Uterus selbst ist grobknotig mit großem, subserösen Knoten, welcher den Douglasschen Raum ausfüllt

Fig. 118. Utérus myomateux avec tumeur ovarienne

Il s'agit d'une tumeur ovarienne cystique, à chambres multiples, intimement soudée à la paroi dorsale de l'utérus. L'utérus même est grossièrement noueux, avec de grands noeuds sousséreux, et remplit le cul-de-sac de Douglas

Fig. 118. Utero miomatoso y tumor de ovario

Se puede observar un tumor de ovario con varios quistes. El tumor se encuentra adherido a la cara posterior del útero. El útero tiene múltiples nódulos, uno de los cuales, el subseroso, es de mayor tamaño y ocupa el fondo de saco posterior (Douglas)

Fig. 118. Utero miomatoso con concomitante tumore ovarico

Si tratta qui di un tumore ovarico cistico e multicamerato, strettamente connesso per aderenze alla parete posteriore dell'utero. L'utero stesso presenta dei grossi noduli miomatosi, come pure dei noduli situati sotto la sierosa. Il cavo del Douglas viene ad essere occupato dai sopracitati noduli

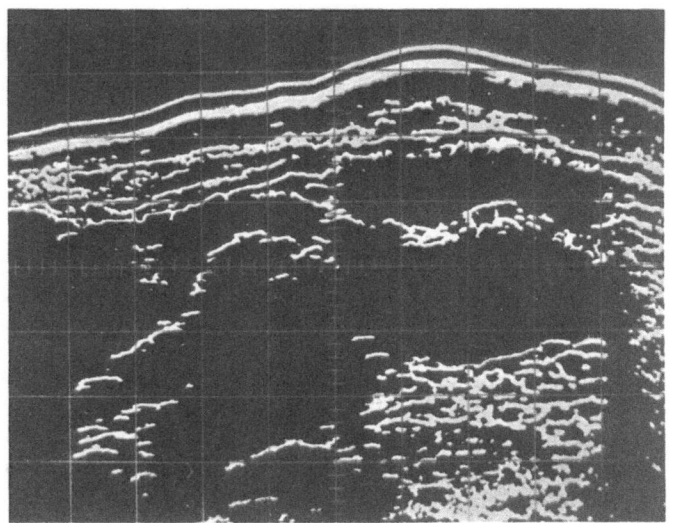

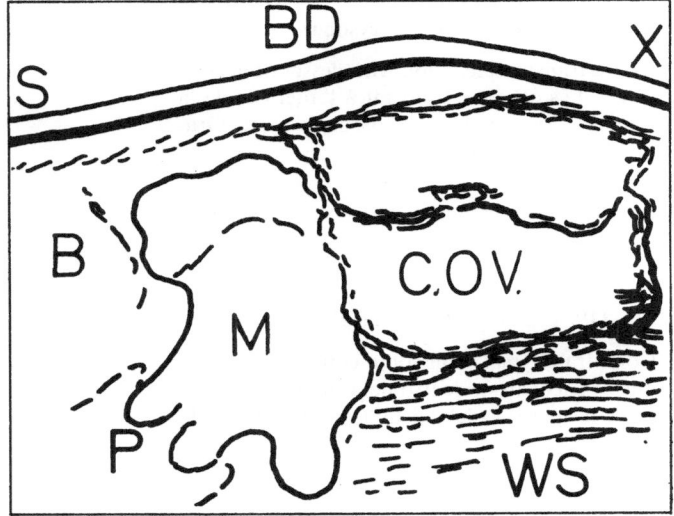

118

Fig. 119. Cystic Ovarian Tumor

Cross section 3-finger widths above the symphysis. The echos in the interior of the tumor
correspond to the wall of the cyst. Scale divisions: 2 cm/section

Abb. 119. Cystischer Ovarialtumor

Querschnitt 3 Querfinger oberhalb der Symphyse. Die Echos, die sich im Inneren des Tumors befinden, entsprechen der Cystenwand.
Skaleneinteilung pro Feld 2 cm

Fig. 119. Tumeur ovarienne cystique

Coupe transversale, 3 doigts au-dessus de la symphyse. Les échos se trouvant à l'intérieur de la
tumeur correspondent à la paroi du kyste. Graduation par champ 2 cm

Fig. 119. Tumor quístico de ovario

Corte transversal 4 cm sobre el pubis. Los ecos
que se encuentran dentro del tumor corresponden a las paredes del quiste. 1 división de escala
= 2 cm

Fig. 119. Tumore cistico ovarico

Sezione condotta 3 dita trasverse al di sopra
della sinfisi pubica. Gli echi trovantesi all'interno della zona occupata dal tumore corrispondono alla parete della cisti. Graduazione della
scala: 2 cm per campo

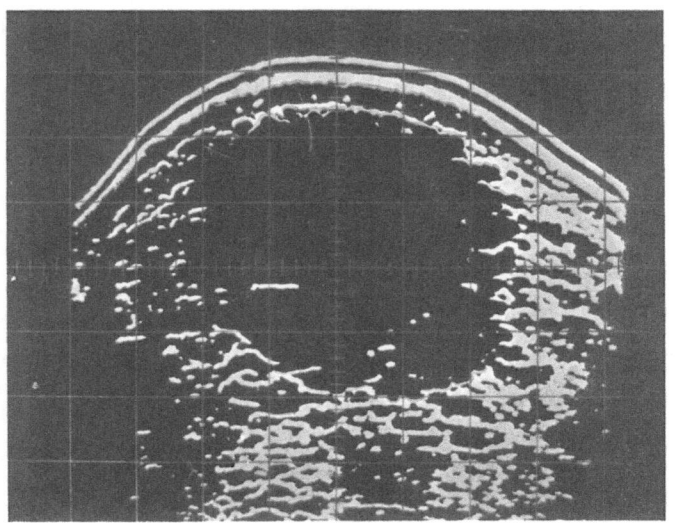

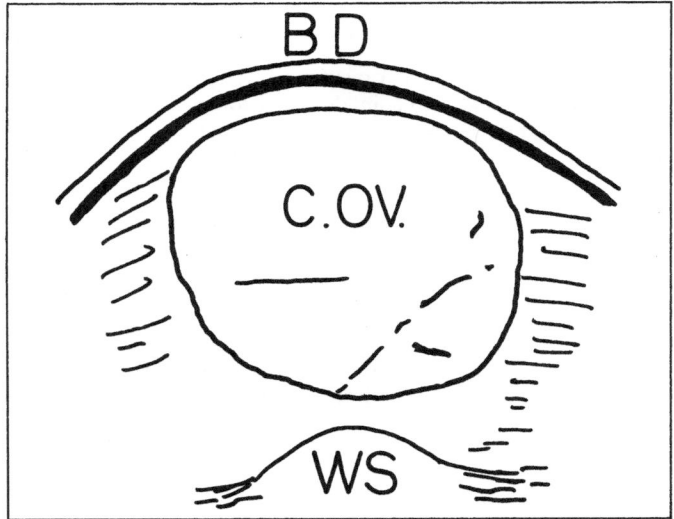

119

Fig. 120. Cystic Ovarian Tumor

Typical picture of a cystic multilocular ovarian tumor. Histologically this is a cystadenoma multiculare mucinosum

Fig. 121. Unilocular Ovarian Tumor

Cross section above the symphysis with a large unilocular ovarian cyst, free of echos. Scale divisions: 2 cm/section

Abb. 120. Cystischer Ovarialtumor

Typisches Bild eines cystischen mehrkammerigen Ovarialtumors. Histologisch handelt es sich um ein Cystadenoma multiculare mucinosum

Abb. 121. Einkammeriger Ovarialtumor

Querschnitt oberhalb der Symphyse bei einer einkammerigen, echoleeren, großen Ovarialcyste. Skaleneinteilung pro Feld 2 cm

Fig. 120. Tumeur ovarienne cystique

Image typique d'une tumeur ovarienne cystique à chambres multiples. Du point de vue histologique, il s'agit d'un cystadenoma multiculare mucinosum

Fig. 121. Tumeur ovarienne simple

Coupe transversale au-dessus de la symphyse d'un grand kyste ovarien simple, exempt d'échos. Graduation par champ 2 cm

Fig. 120. Tumor quístico de ovario

Se puede observar un tumor de ovario de varios quistes. Histológicamente se trata de un cistoadenoma mucinoso

Fig. 121. Tumor de ovario de un solo quiste

Corte transversal suprapúbico. Se puede observar el quiste con la zona libre de ecos. 1 división de escala = 2 cm

Fig. 120. Tumore ovarico cistico

Aspetto tipico di un tumore cistico all'ovaio (multicamerato). Istologicamente si tratta di un cistoadenoma multiloculare mucinoso

Fig. 121. Tumore ovarico ad una sola cavità

Sezione condotta al di sopra della sinfisi pubica. Grossa cisti ovarica ad una sola cavità, senza eco. Graduazione della scala: 2 cm per campo

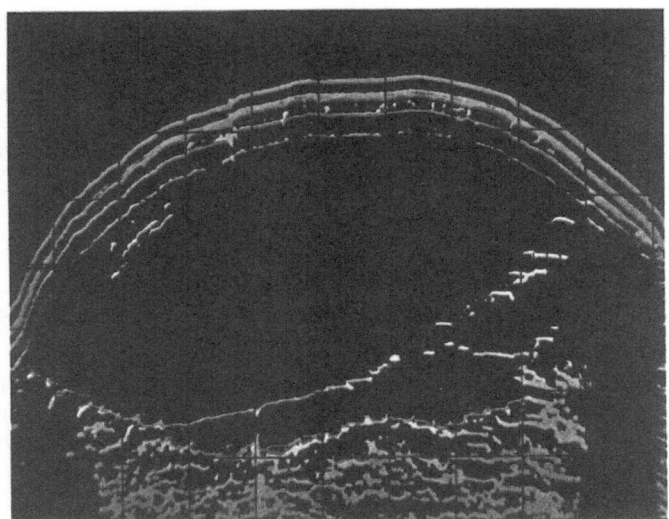

120

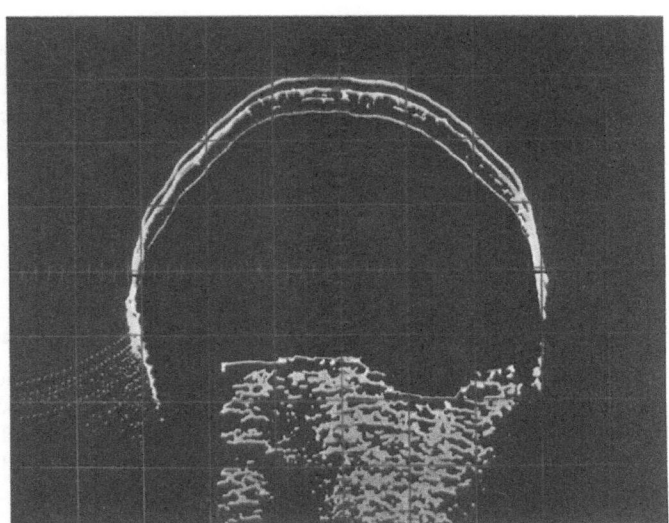

121

Fig. 122. Multilocular Ovarian Tumor

Cross section above the symphysis with a multi-locular ovarian tumor. Inside the tumor, a few echo structures that which originate from the cyst walls, can be seen. Scale divisions: 1 cm/section

Fig. 123. Multilocular Ovarian Tumor

Longitudinal section in the same case as Fig. 122. The bladder can be seen below the tumor. Here the scale divisions are 2 cm/section. Sound frequency: 2 MHz

Abb. 122. Mehrkammeriger Ovarialtumor

Querschnitt oberhalb der Symphyse bei einem mehrkammerigen Ovarialtumor. Innerhalb des Tumors sind einige Echostrukturen zu erkennen, die von den Cystenwänden ausgehen. Skaleneinteilung pro Feld 1 cm

Abb. 123. Mehrkammeriger Ovarialtumor

Längsschnitt bei gleichem Fall wie Abb. 122. Caudal vom Tumor ist die Harnblase zu erkennen. Hier beträgt die Skaleneinteilung pro Feld 2 cm. Schallfrequenz 2 MHZ

Fig. 122. Tumeur ovarienne à chambres multiples

Coupe transversale au-dessus de la symphyse d'une tumeur ovarienne à chambres multiples. A l'intérieur de la tumeur on aperçoit quelques structures d'échos, provenant des parois de kyste. Graduation par champ 1 cm

Fig. 123. Tumeur ovarienne à chambres multiples

Coupe longitudinale du même cas que l'image 122. On aperçoit la vessie en direction caudale de la tumeur. La graduation par champ mesure ici 2 cm. Fréquence de son 2 MHz

Fig. 122. Tumor de ovario de quistes múltiples

Corte transversal suprapúbico. Los ecos en el tumor provienen de reflejos de los tabiques. 1 división de escala = 1 cm

Fig. 123. Tumor de ovario de quistes múltiples

Mismo caso de la figura anterior. Corte longitudinal. En dirección caudal del tumor se encuentra la vejiga. 1 división de escala = 2 cm. Frecuencia del ultrasonido = 2 MHz

Fig. 122. Tumore ovarico a piu' cavità

Sezione condotta al di sopra della sinfisi in caso di tumore ovarico multicavitario. Nell'interno del tumore si possono riconoscere alcune strutture dovute agli echi provenienti dalle pareti cistiche. Graduazione della scala: 1 cm per campo

Fig. 123. Tumore ovarico multicavitario

Sezione longitudinale, caso uguale alla Fig. 122. Caudalmente al tumore si riconosce la vescica urinaria. Graduazione della scala: 2 cm per campo. Frequenza: 2 MHZ

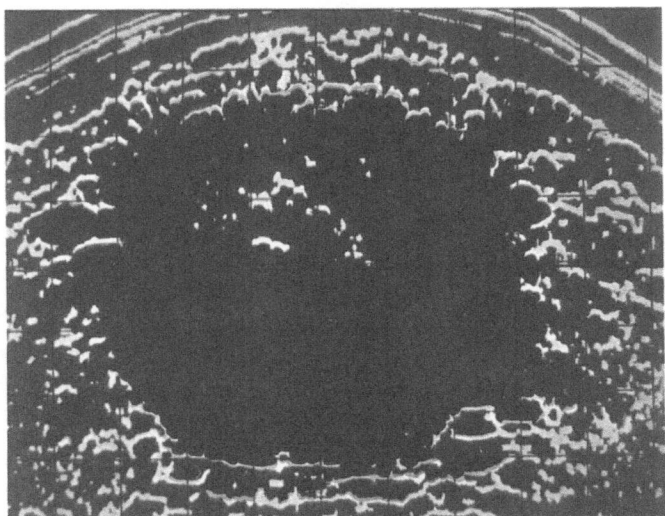

122

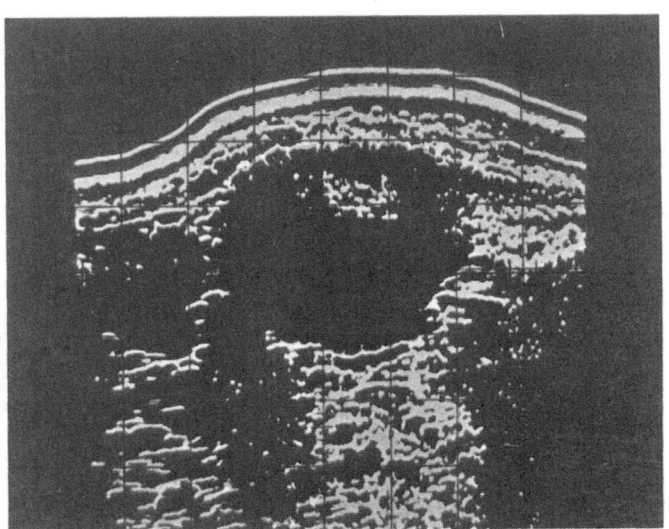

123

Fig. 124. Ovarian Carcinoma

Longitudinal section in the median line with an ovarian carcinoma. Distinct structures are to be seen within the tumor. Histologically this is a papillary cystadenocarcinoma

Fig. 125. Ovarian Carcinoma

Cross section between symphysis and navel; same case as Fig. 124. Scale divisions are 2 cm/section and sound frequency is 2 MHz

Abb. 124. Ovarialcarcinom

Längsschnitt in der Medianlinie bei einem Ovarialcarcinom. Innerhalb des Tumors sind deutliche Strukturen zu erkennen. Histologisch handelt sich um ein papilläres Cystadenocarcinom

Abb. 125. Ovarialcarcinom

Querschnitt zwischen Symphyse und Nabel, gleicher Fall wie Abb. 124. Skaleneinteilung beträgt pro Feld 2 cm und Schallfrequenz 2 MHZ

Fig. 124. Carcinome ovarien

Coupe longitudinale dans la ligne médiane d'un carcinome ovarien. On aperçoit des structures distinctes à l'intérieur de la tumeur. Du point de vue histologique, il s'agit d'un cyst-adénocarcinome papillaire

Fig. 125. Carcinome ovarien

Coupe transversale entre le nombril et la symphyse. Même cas que l'image 124. Graduation par champ 2 cm. Fréquence de son 2 MHz

Fig. 124. Tumor de ovario

Corte longitudinal en línea media. Dentro del tumor se pueden observar múltiples ecos. Histológicamente se trata de un cistoadenocarcinoma

Fig. 125. Tumor de ovario

Mismo caso de la figura anterior. Corte transversal a media distancia del pubis y ombligo. 1 división de escala = 2 cm. Frecuencia del ultrasonido = 2 MHz

Fig. 124. Carcinoma ovarico

Sezione longitudinale condotta sulla linea mediana di un carcinoma ovarico. Nell'interno del tumore sono chiaramente riconoscibili delle strutture. Istologicamente si tratta di un cistoadenocarcinoma papillifero

Fig. 125. Carcinoma ovarico

Sezione condotta attraverso la sinfisi e l'ombelico, caso uguale alla Fig. 124. Graduazione di scala: 2 cm. per campo. Frequenza 2 MHZ

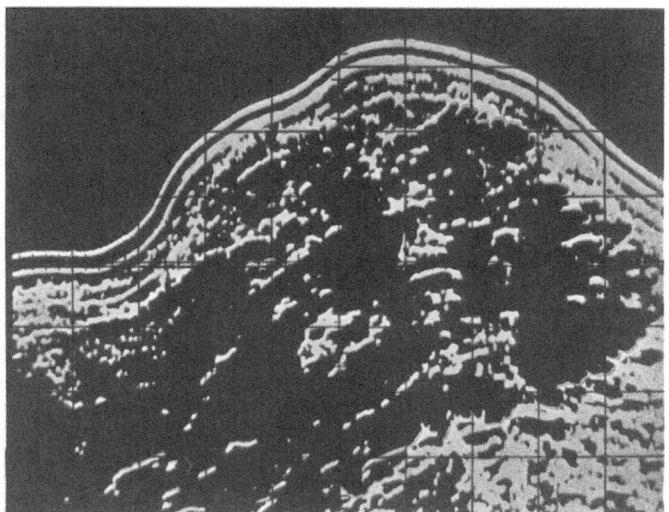

124

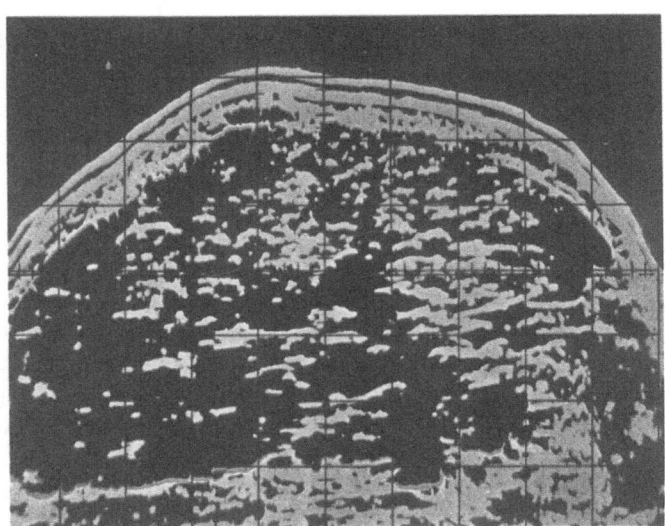

125

Fig. 126. Ovarian Carcinoma

Longitudinal section in the median line with a solid ovarian tumor (Carcinoma). Structures can be seen within the tumor. Below the tumor is the uterus in a state of anteflexion

Fig. 127. Ovarian Carcinoma

Cross section 2-finger widths below the navel in the same case as Fig. 126. Scale divisions are 2 cm/section and sound frequency is 2 MHz

Abb. 126. Ovarialcarcinom

Längsschnitt in der Medianlinie bei einem soliden Ovarialtumor (Carcinom). Innerhalb des Tumors sind Strukturen zu erkennen. Caudal vom Tumor liegt der Uterus in anteflektiertem Zustand

Abb. 127. Ovarialcarcinom

Querschnitt 2 Querfinger unterhalb des Nabels bei gleichem Fall wie Abb. 126. Skaleneinteilung beträgt pro Feld 2 cm und Schallfrequenz 2 MHZ

Fig. 126. Carcinome ovarien

Coupe longitudinale dans la ligne médiane d'une tumeur ovarienne solide (carcinome). On aperçoit des structures à l'intérieur de la tumeur. L'utérus, en état d'antéflexion, se trouve en direction caudale de la tumeur

Fig. 127. Carcinome ovarien

Coupe transversale, 2 doigts en-dessous du nombril. Même cas que l'image 126. Graduation par champ 2 cm. Fréquence de son 2 MHz

Fig. 126. Tumor de ovario

Corte longitudinal en línea media. Se observa un tumor sólido de ovario que histológicamente corresponde a un carcinoma. El útero se encuentra en anteversoflexión

Fig. 127. Tumor de ovario

Mismo caso de la figura anterior. Corte transversal a 2 cm. sobre el pubis. 1 división de escala = 2 cm. Frecuencia del ultrasonido = 2 MHz

Fig. 126. Carcinoma ovarico

Sezione longitudinale condotta sulla linea mediana. Caso di tumore ovariale solido (carcinoma). All'interno del tumore sono riconoscibili alcune strutture. Caudalmente al tumore si trova l'utero in posizione anteflessa

Fig. 127. Carcinoma ovarico

Sezione condotta 2 dita trasverse al di sotto dell'ombelico. Caso uguale alla Fig. 126. Graduazione di scala 2 cm per campo. Frequenza 2 MHZ

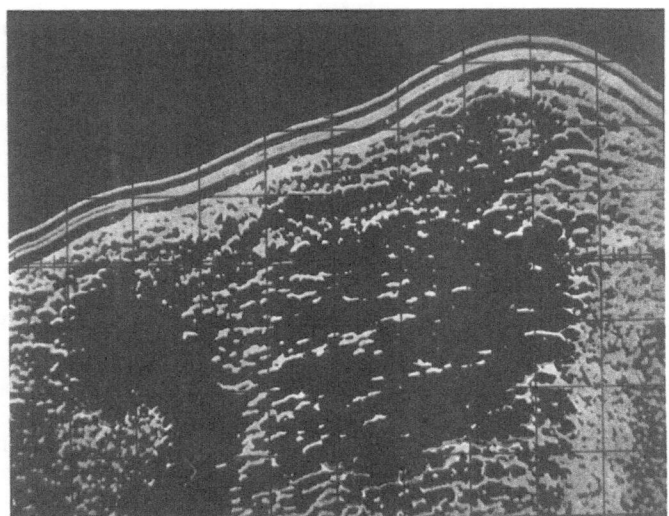

126

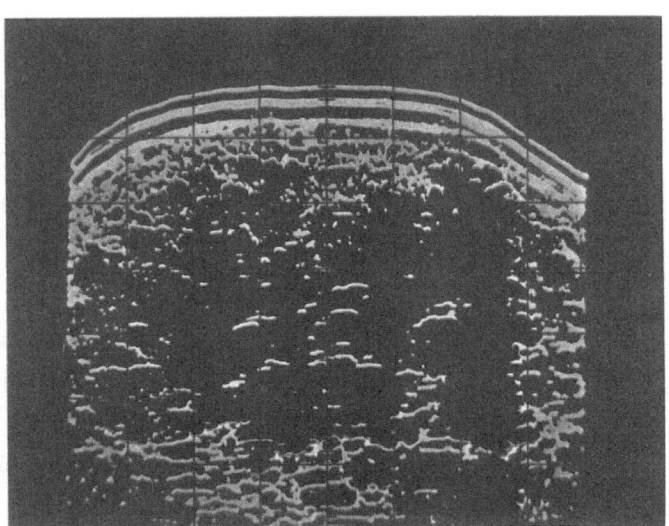

127

Pregnancy with Uterine Myoma

Gravidität bei Uterus myomatosus
Grossesse et utérus myomateux
Embrazo y útero miomatoso
Utero miomatoso in gravidanza

Fig. 128. Pregnancy with Uterine Myoma

Longitudinal section in the median line. There is a uterine myoma with subserosal myomic nodules on the anterior wall of the uterus, and also a large cervical myoma. In the center, the fetal head can be seen, in the 22nd week

Abb. 128. Gravidität bei Uterus myomatosus

Längsschnitt in der Medianlinie. Es besteht ein Uterus myomatosus mit subserösen Myomknoten an der Uterusvorderwand sowie ein großes Cervixmyom. In der Mitte ist der kindliche Kopf in der 22. Woche sichtbar

Fig. 128. Grossesse d'un utérus myomateux

Coupe longitudinale dans la ligne médiane. Il existe un utérus myomateux avec des noeuds myomateux sous-séreux à la paroi ventrale de l'utérus, ainsi qu'un grand myome du col de l'utérus. On aperçoit au milieu la tête d'enfant dans la 22ᵉ semaine

Fig. 128. Embarazo y útero miomatoso

Corte longitudinal en línea media. Mioma subseroso en cara anterior del útero y mioma cervical. En el centro se observa la cabeza fetal. 22 semanas de gestación

Fig. 128. Utero miomatoso in gravidanza

Sezione longitudinale sulla linea mediana. Si nota la oresenza di un mioma uterino, con noduli sottosierosi sulla parete anteriore, come pure la presenza di un grosso mioma cervicale. Nel mezzo si nota la testa del feto (22a settimana di gravidanza)

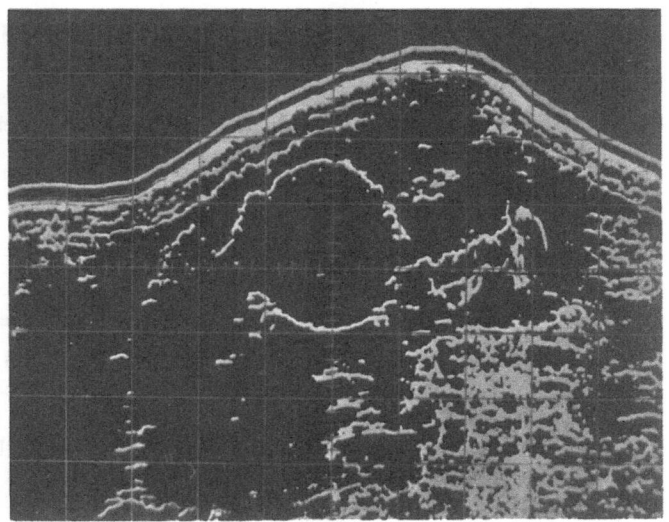

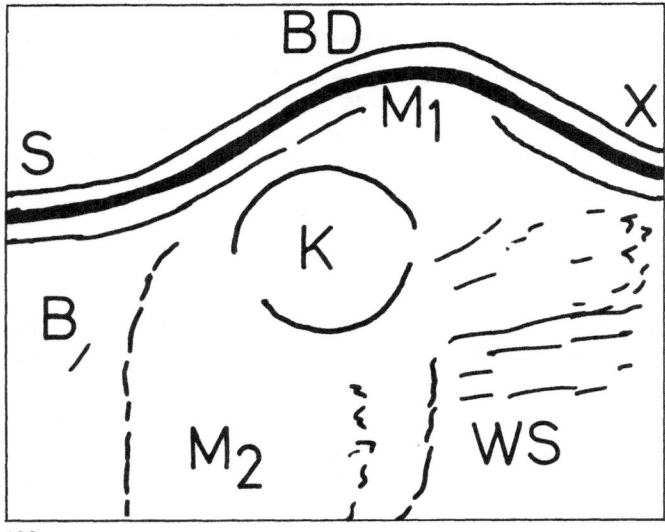

128

Fig. 129. Uterine Myoma in the 22nd Week of Pregnancy

Longitudinal section to the left of the median line; same case as Fig. 128. Here, small parts and the cervical myoma are visible. The bladder is below

Fig. 130. Uterine Myoma in the 22nd Week

Same case as Fig. 129, but cross section above the symphysis. The cervix and cervical myoma are visible behind the bladder. Scale divisions: 2 cm/section

Abb. 129. Uterus myomatosus in der 22. Woche

Längsschnitt links von der Medianlinie, gleicher Fall wie Abb. 128, hier sind kleine Teile und das Cervixmyom sichtbar. Caudal liegt Harnblase

Abb. 130. Uterus myomatosus in der 22. Woche

Gleicher Fall wie Abb. 129, jedoch suprasymphysärer Querschnitt. Hinter der Blase sind die Cervix und das Cervixmyom sichtbar. Skaleneinteilung pro Feld 2 cm

Fig. 129. Utérus myomateux dans la 22e semaine

Coupe longitudinale à gauche de la ligne médiane. Même cas que l'image 128. Ici, des parties foetales et le myome du col sont visibles. La vessie se trouve en direction caudale

Fig. 130. Utérus myomateux dans la 22e semaine

Même cas que l'image 129, mais en coupe transversale suprasymphysaire. On aperçoit le col de l'utérus et le myome du col derrière la vessie. Graduation par champ 2 cm

Fig. 129. Embarazo y útero miomatoso — 22 semanas de gestación

Mismo caso de la figura 128. Corte longitudinal a la izquierda de la línea media. Se pueden observar extremidades fetales y el mioma cervical. En dirección caudal se encuentra la vejiga

Fig. 130. Embarazo y útero miomatoso — 22 semanas de gestación

Mismo caso de la figura 129. Corte transversal suprapúbico. Detrás de la vejiga se puede observar el cuello uterino y el mioma cervical. 1 división de escala = 2 cm

Fig. 129. Utero miomatoso nella 22a settimana di gravidanza

Sezione longitudinale a sinistra della linea mediana, caso uguale alla Fig. 128. Qui sono visibili le piccole parti fetali come il mioma cervicale. Caudalmente si vede la vescica

Fig. 130. Utero miomatoso nella 22a settimana di gravidanza

Caso uguale alle Fig. 129, con. Sezione soprasinfisaria. Dietro la vescica urinaria é visibile il canale cervicale e il mioma cervicale. Graduazione della scala 2 cm per campo

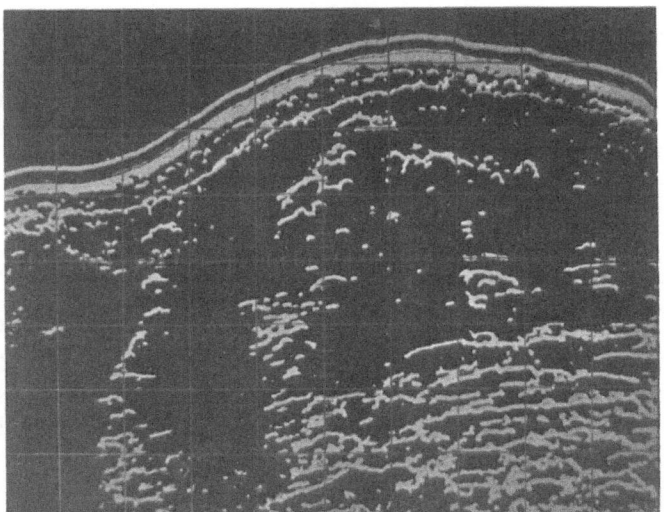

129

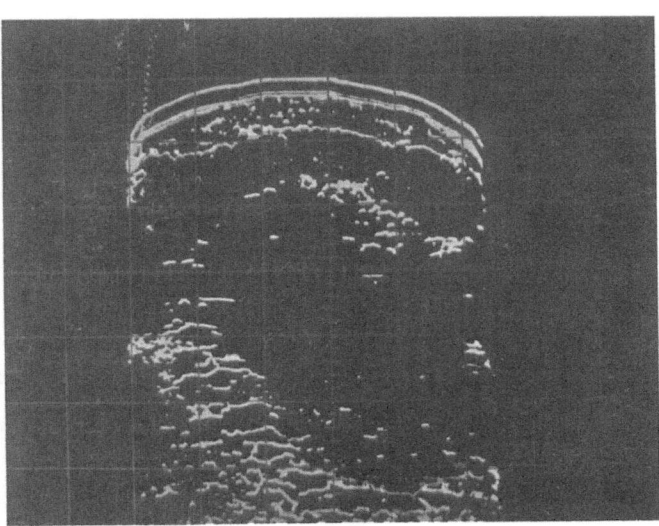

130

Ultrasonic Diagnosis on the Upper Abdomen

Ultraschalldiagnostik am Oberbauch
Diagnostic à ultrasons dans l'épigastre
Diagnóstico ultrasónico en abdomen
L'ecografia diagnostica nella parte superiore dell' addome

Fig. 131. Both Kidneys in Cross Section

Sub-costal cross section in the prone position. Left and right kidneys of equal size. Scale divisions: 3 cm/section

Abb. 131. Beide Nieren im Querschnitt

Subcostaler Querschnitt in Bauchlage. Linke und rechte Niere gleichgroß. Skaleneinteilung pro Feld 3 cm

Fig. 131. Les deux reins en coupe transversale

Coupe transversale sous-costale en position ventrale. Les reins droit et gauche sont de même grandeur. Graduation par champ 3 cm

Fig. 131. Corte transversal de ambos riñones

Corte transversal subcostal. Ambos riñones de igual tamaño. 1 división de escala = 3 cm

Fig. 131. Reni in sezione trasversale

Sezione subcostale in posizione sul ventre. I due reni presentano un'eguale grandezza. Graduazione di scala: 3 cm per campo

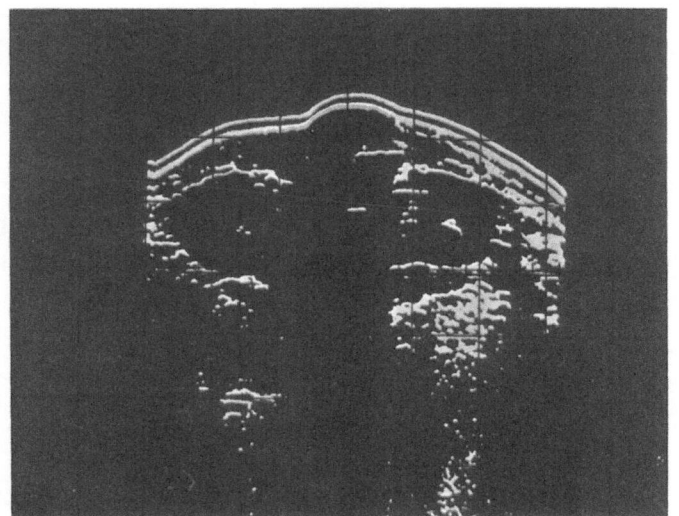

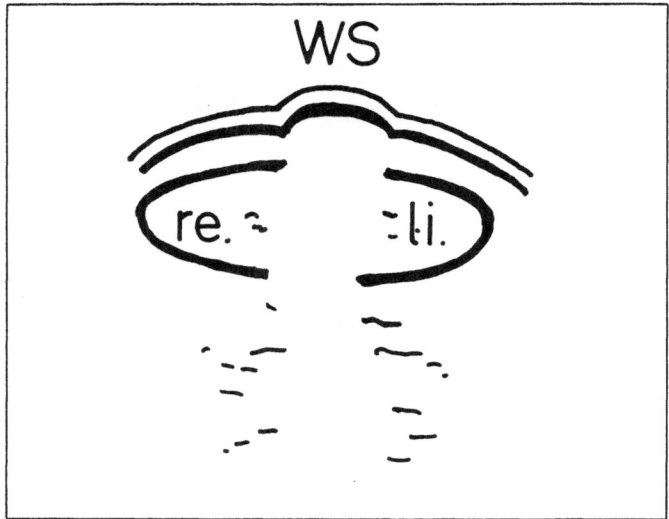

131

Fig. 132. Both Kidneys in Cross Section

Same case as Fig. 131; both kidneys of equal size;
scale divisions here are 2 cm/section

Abb. 132. Beide Nieren im Querschnitt

Gleicher Fall wie Abb. 131, beide Nieren gleichgroß. Skaleneinteilung pro Feld hier 2 cm

Fig. 132. Les deux reins en coupe transversale

Même cas que l'image 131. Deux reins de même
grandeur. La graduation par champ mesure ici
2 cm

Fig. 132. Corte transversal de ambos riñones

Mismo caso de la figura 131. 1 división de
escala = 2 cm

Fig. 132. Ambedue i reni in sezione trasversale

Caso uguale alla Fig. 131, i due reni sono di
eguale grandezza. Graduazione della scala: 2 cm
per campo

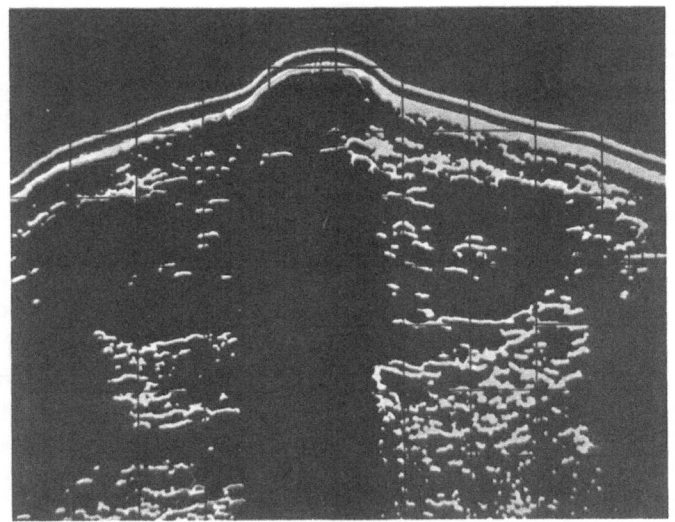

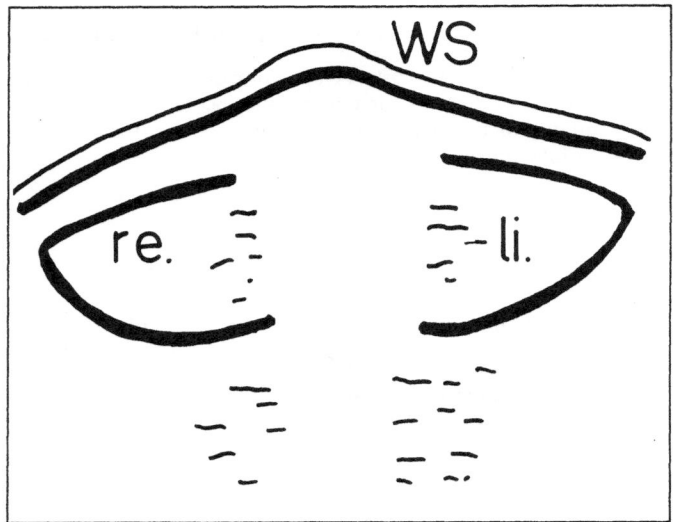

132

Fig. 133. Both Kidneys in Cross Section

Sub-costal cross section in the prone position. Here the right kidney is distinctly smaller than the left. This finding was subsequently confirmed by radiography

Fig. 134. Both Kidneys in Cross Section

Same case as Fig. 133. Here again the reduced size of the right kidney is clearly recognisable. Scale divisions: 2 cm/section

Abb. 133. Beide Nieren im Querschnitt

Subcostaler Querschnitt in Bauchlage. Hier ist die rechte Niere eindeutig kleiner als die linke. Dieser Befund wurde anschließend röntgenologisch bestätigt

Abb. 134. Beide Nieren im Querschnitt

Gleicher Fall wie Abb. 133. Hier ist ebenfalls die verkleinerte rechte Niere gut zu erkennen. Skaleneinteilung pro Feld 2 cm

Fig. 133. Les deux reins en coupe transversale

Coupe transversale sous-costale en position dorsale. Ici, le rein droit est nettement plus petit que celui de gauche. Ce constat fut ensuite confirmé radiologiquement

Fig. 134. Les deux reins en coupe transversale

Même cas que l'image 133. Ici également, on perçoit nettement le rein droit rapetissé. Graduation par champ 2 cm

Fig. 133. Corte transversal de ambos riñones

Corte transversal subcostal. El riñón derecho es menor que el izquierdo, lo que posteriormente fué comprobado por radiologia

Fig. 134. Corte transversal de ambos riñones

Mismo caso de la figura anterior. Se puede observar que el riñón derecho es menor que el izquierdo. 1 división de escala = 2 cm

Fig. 133. Reni in sezione subcostale

Sezione subcostale in posizione orizzontale sull'addome. In questo caso si vede come il rene di destra sia piu' piccolo di quello di sinistra. Questo risultato venne confermato piu' tardi per via radiografica

Fig. 134. Reni in sezione trasversale

Caso uguale alla Fig. 133. Anche qui si riconosce bene come il rene di destra sia piu' piccolo di quello di sinistra. Graduazione della scala: 2 cm

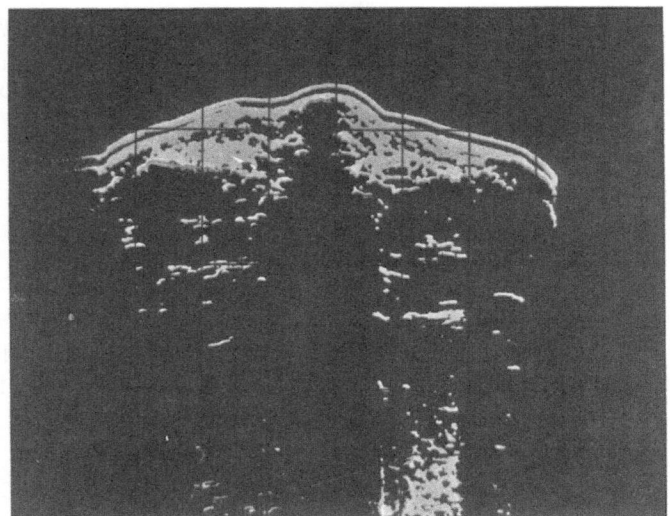

133

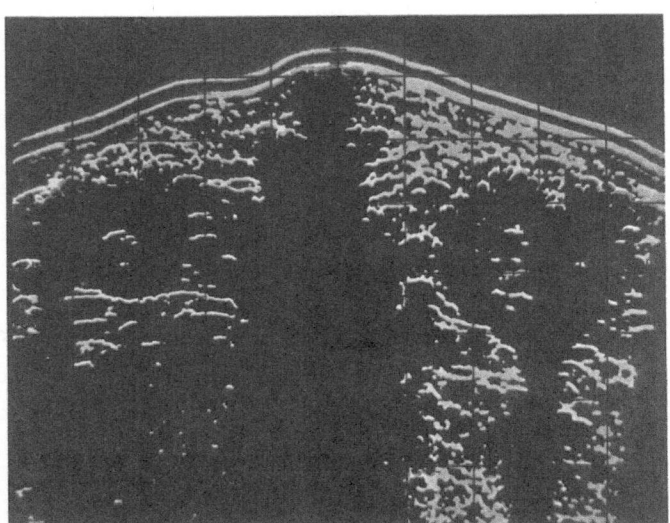

134

Fig. 135. Hydronephrosis, Right

Sub-costal cross section in the prone position. There is a pronounced hydronephrosis of the right kidney. Scale division/section: 3 cm

Fig. 136. Pronounced Hydronephrosis, Right

Same picture as Fig. 135, but with scale divisions of 2 cm/section

Abb. 135. Hydronephrose rechts

Subcostaler Querschnitt in Bauchlage. Es handelt sich um eine ausgeprägte Hydronephrose der rechten Niere. Skaleneinteilung pro Feld 3 cm

Abb. 136. Ausgeprägte Hydronephrose rechts

Gleiches Bild wie Abb. 135, jedoch mit Skaleneinteilung pro Feld 2 cm

Fig. 135. Hydronéphrose droite

Coupe transversale sous-costale en position ventrale. Il s'agit d'une hydronéphrose marquée du rein droit. Graduation par champ 3 cm

Fig. 136. Hydronéphrose marquée droite

Même image que l'image 135, mais avec une graduation par champ de 2 cm

Fig. 135. Hidronefrosis derecha

Corte transversal subcostal en decúbito prono. Se puede observar la hidronefrosis del riñón derecho. 1 división de escala = 3 cm

Fig. 136. Hidronefrosis derecha

Mismo caso de la figura anterior. 1 división de escala = 2 cm

Fig. 135. Idronefrosi destra

Sezione subcostale in posizione sul ventre. Si tratta di una forte idronefrosi del rene destro. Graduazione della scala: 3 cm per campo

Fig. 136. Idronefrosi destra

Caso uguale alla Fig. 135. Graduazione della scala: 2 cm per campo

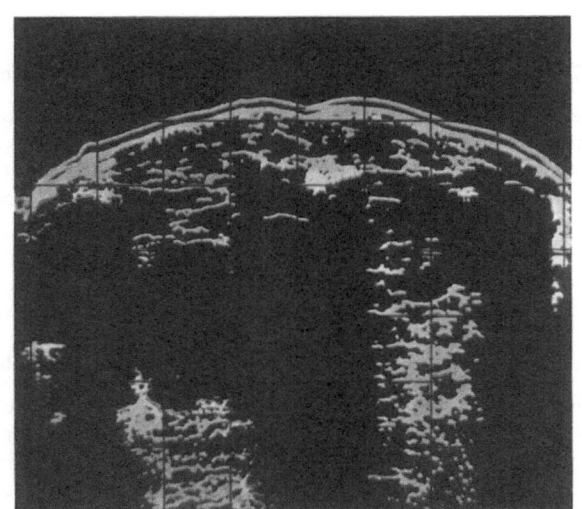

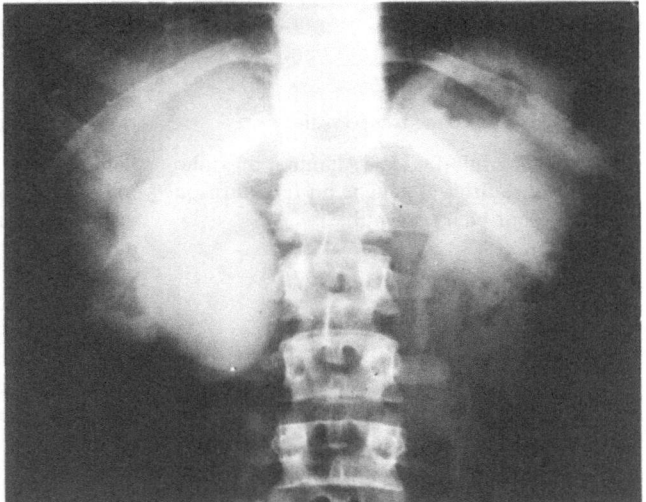

135

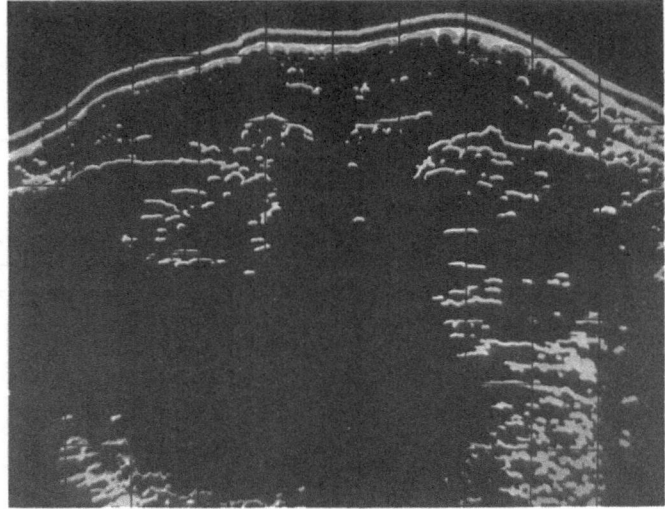

136

Fig. 137. Liver in Cross Section

Cross section of a liver at the level of the xiphoid. Left and right lobes of liver and stomach are clearly recognisable

Fig. 138. Liver in Cross Section

Cross section, also at the level of the xiphoid. There are small echos inside the liver; it is highly probable that these are due to metastases. Scale divisions: 3 cm/section

Abb. 137. Leber im Querschnitt

Querschnitt einer Leber auf der Höhe des Xiphoides. Rechter und linker Leberlappen sowie Magen gut zu erkennen

Abb. 138. Leber im Querschnitt

Querschnitt ebenfalls auf Höhe der Xiphoides. Innerhalb der Leber sind kleine Echos. Mit sehr großer Wahrscheinlichkeit könnte es sich um Metastasen handeln. Skaleneinteilung pro Feld 3 cm

Fig. 137. Foie en coupe transversale

Coupe transversale d'un foie à hauteur du xiphoïde. Les lobes droit et gauche du foie ainsi que l'estomac sont bien perceptibles

Fig. 138. Foie en coupe transversale

Coupe transversale, également à hauteur du xiphoïde. A l'intérieur du foie, il y a de petits échos. Il s'agit très probablement de métastases. Graduation par champ 3 cm

Fig. 137. Corte transversal del hígado a nivel de xifoides

Se puede observar el lóbulo derecho e izquierdo del hígado, asi como el estómago

Fig. 138. Corte transversal del hígado a nivel de xifoides

En la imagen del hígado se pueden observar ecos que muy probablemente son debidos a metástasis. 1 división de escala = 3 cm

Fig. 137. Fegato in sezione trasversale

Sezione trasversale del fegato condotta a livello del processo xifoide. Si riconoscono i lobi epatici destro e sinistro, come pure lo stomaco

Fig. 138. Fegato in sezione trasversale

Sezione trasversale condotta anche in questo caso a livello del processo xifoide. Nel mezzo del parenchima epatico vi sono piccoli echi. Molto probabilmente si tratta qui di una metastasi. Graduazione di scala: 3 cm per campo

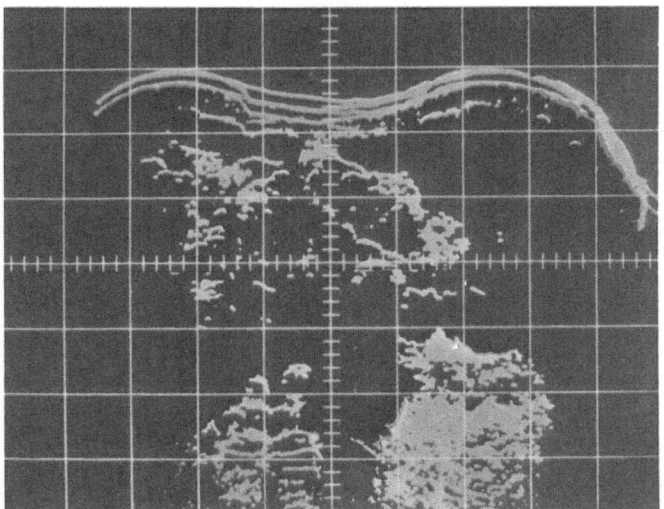

137

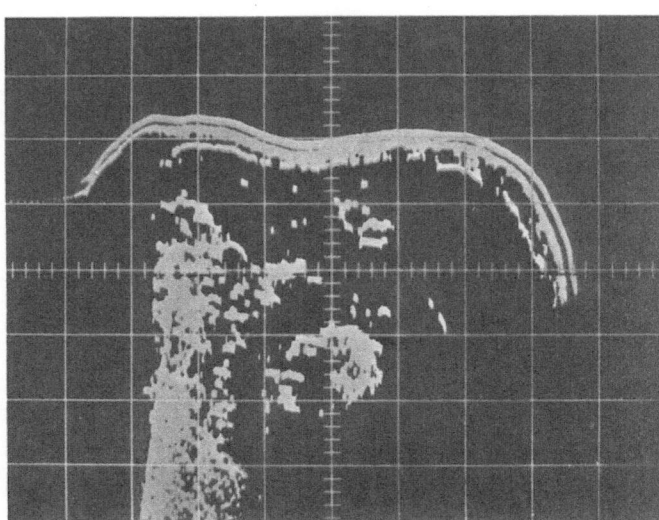

138

References

ADLER, U., GRUENINGER, B.: Über die Zuverlässigkeit der röntgenologischen Messungen des Fetus in utero. Gynaecologia (Basel) **147**, 522 (1959).

AIERS, M., EVERED, D.C., SMITH, A.H.: Placental localization by the use of 132-J-Human Serum Albumin and by ultrasonic scanning. A comparative Study. J. Obstet. Gynaec. Brit. Cwlth **76**, 220 (1969).

ALBRECHT, K.F., HAULEN, H., DAVEDTS, H.H., KRAUSE, K.: Ultraschalluntersuchung bei Tumoren und Cysten an der Niere. Helv. chir. Acta **38**, 509 (1971).

ALTH, G.: Beitrag zur Lokalisationstechnik bei gynäkologischer Tiefenbestrahlung. Strahlentherapie **137**, 649 (1969).

ALTH, G., KRATOCHWIL, A., HOFNER, W.: Zur Herdsuche in der gynäkologischen Strahlentherapie. Strahlentherapie **142**, 303 (1971).

ASHER, W.M.: Echographic diagnosis of retroperitoneal lymphnode enlargement. Ultrasound scanning technique and diagnostic findings. Amer. J. Roentgenol. **195**, 438 (1969).

BAUCH, U.: Die Schätzung von Länge und Gewicht aus verschiedenen Körpermassen des Neugeborenen im Hinblick auf die intrauterine Untersuchung. Inaug.-Diss., Münster 1972.

BEAZLEY, J.M., MATHEWS, J.C., LEAVER, E.P.: Placental localization using 99 m-Technetium labelled serum albumin. J. Obstet. Gynaec. Brit. Cwlth **75**, 470 (1968).

BOOG, G., MOT, E. DE, MULLER, G., KUHN, A., GANDAR, R.: Le diagnostic ultrasonique des tumeurs pelviennes. Rev. franç. Gynéc. **65**, 679 (1970).

BORELL, U., FERNSTROEM, J., OHLSEN, L.: The halo sign in the living and dead fetus. Amer. J. Obstet. Gynec. **87**, 906 (1963).

BREGULLA, K., RETTENMAIER, G., RUMMEL, W.D., KROENERT, E.: Der Wert der Ultraschalluntersuchung bei der Differentialdiagnose zwischen einer Gravidität bei einem Uterus myomatosus und einer Blasenmole. Geburtsh. u. Frauenheilk. **30**, 1116 (1970).

CAMPBELL, S.: Ultrasonic fetal cephalometry during the second trimester of pregnancy. J. Obstet. Gynaec. Brit. Cwlth **77**, 1057 (1970).

CRICHTON, D.: The accuracy of X-ray cephalometry in utero. Proc. roy. Soc. Med. **45**, 535 (1952).

DAMASCELLI, B., BONADONNA, G., MUSUMECI, R., LENTHI, C.U.: Two dimensional pulsed echodetection of paraaortic lymphnodes. Surg. Gynec. Obstet. **128**, 772 (1969).

DONALD, I.: Use of ultrasonics in diagnosis of abdominal swellings. Brit. med. J. **1963 I** 1154.

DONALD, I.: Ultrasonic echo sounding in obstetrical and gynecological diagnosis. Amer. J. Obstet. Gynec. **93**, 935 (1965).

DONALD, I.: The interpretation of abdominal ultrasonograms. In: Diagnostic ultrasound. Hrsg.: Grossmann, C.C., J.H. Holmes, C. Joynes, E.W. Purnell, p. 316. New York: Plenum-Press 1966.

DONALD, I.: Ultrasonics in obstetrics. Brit. med. Bull. **24**, 71 (1968).

DONALD, I., ABDULLA, U.: Ultrasonics in obstetrics and gynaecology. Brit. J. Radiol. **40**, 604 (1967).

DONALD, I., MAC VICAR, J., BROWN, T.G.: Investigation of abdominal masses by pulsed ultrasound. Lancet **1958 I**, 1188.

GRUENWALD, P.: Growth of the human fetus. I. Normal growth and its variation. Amer. J. Obstet. Gynec. **94**, 1112 (1966).

GRUENWALD, P.: Growth in the human fetus. II. Abnormal growths in twins and infants of mothers with diabetes, hypertension or isoimmunization. Amer. J. Obstet. Gynec. **94**, 1120 (1966).

HANSMANN, M., BÄKER, H., FABULA, ST., MÜLLER-SCHOLTES, H., NELLEN, H.J., VOIGT, U.: Biometrische Daten des Feten — Ergebnisse einer modifizierten Methodik der Ultraschall-Diagnostik. In: Perinatale Medizin, Bd. III. Ed.: Saling, E. u. J.W. Dudenhausen. Stuttgart: Thieme 1972.

HAUBOLD, U.: Plazenta-Lokalisation mit Radioisotopen. Visum **1**, 19 (1969).

HELLMANN, L.M., KOBAYASHI, M., FILLISTI, L., LAVENHAR, M.: Sources of error in sonographic fetal mesuration and estimation of growth. Amer. J. Obstet. Gynec. **99**, 662 (1967).

HERNANDY, T., NEUBAUER, G.: Isotopenplacentographie. Fortschr. Röntgenstr. **109**, 4 (1968).

HICKL, E.-J., DELUCCA, A., HAUBOLD, U.: Vergleichende Untersuchungen über Plazentalokalisation mit Ultraschall und radioaktiven Isotopen. Geburtsh. u. Frauenheilk. **30**, 316 (1970).

HINSELMANN, M.: Die praktische Bedeutung der Ultraschalldiagnostik in der Geburtshilfe. Gynaecologia (Basel) **165**, 127–130 (1968).

HINSELMANN, M.: Ein neues Ultraschall-Schnittbildgerät und seine praktische Anwendungsmöglichkeit in der Geburtshilfe. Gynaecologia (Basel) **167**, 303 (1969).

HINSELMANN, M.: Ultraschalldiagnostik in der Geburtshilfe. Gynäkologe **2**, 45 (1969).

HINSELMANN, M.: Ultraschalldiagnostik in der Geburtshilfe. Dtsch. med. Wschr. **94**, 316 (1969).

HOBSON, B.M.: Further observations on the excretion of chorionic gonadotrophin by women hydatidiform mole. J. Obstet. Gynaec. Brit. Emp. **65**, 253 (1958).

HODGES, P.C.: Roentgen pelvimetry and fetometry. Amer. J. Roentgenol. **37**, 644 (1937).

HOFFBAUER, H.: Über die Ultraschalldiagnostik der Plazenta. In: Saling, E., K.A. Hüter, Fortschritte der perinatalen Medizin. Stuttgart: Thieme 1971.

HOFMANN, D.: Neue Möglichkeiten der Ultraschalldiagnostik in der Gynäkologie und Geburtshilfe. Fortschr. Med. **84**, 689 (1966).

HOFMANN, D., HOLLAENDER, H.-J.: Die Anwendung des Ultraschallschnittbildgerätes VIDOSON in der Gynäkologie und Geburtshilfe. Electromedica **4**, 105 (1968).

HOFMANN, D., HOLLAENDER, H.J.: Die intrauterine Diagnostik des Hydrops fetus universalis mittels Ultraschall. Zbl. Gynäk. **90**, 667 (1968).

HOFMANN, D., HOLLAENDER, H.J., WEISER, P.: Über die geburtshilfliche Bedeutung der Ultraschalldiagnostik. Gynaecologia **164**, 24 (1967).

HOHLWEG, W.: Die diagnostische Bedeutung der immunologischen Kontrolle der Gonadotropinausscheidung im Harn. Wien. med. Wschr. **118**, 804 (1968).

HOLM, H.H., MORTENSEN, T.: Ultrasonic scanning in diagnosis of abdominal disease. Acta chir. scand. **134**, 333 (1968).

HOLM, H.H., RASMUSSEN, S.N., KRISTENSEN, J.K.: Identification of ultrasonic pictures of the abdomen. Ultrasonics **9**, 49 (1971).

HOLLAENDER, H.J.: Nachweis und Differentialdiagnostik intraabdominaler Tumoren mittels Ultraschall. Med. Klin. **63**, 1175 (1968).

HOLLAENDER, H.J.: Die Ultraschall-Diagnostik in der Schwangerschaft. München-Berlin-Wien: Urban & Schwarzenberg 1972.

HOLLAENDER, H.J., MAST, H.: Intrauterine Dikkenmessung der Plazenta mittels Ultraschall bei normalen Schwangerschaften und bei Rhesus-Inkompatibilität. Geburtsh. u. Frauenheilk. **28**, 626 (1968).

HOLTORFF, J.: Über die kindliche Mortalität bei Zwillingsgeburten. Zbl. Gynäk. **86**, 1529 (1964).

HOSEMANN, H.: Schwangerschaftsdauer und Kopfumfang des Neugeborenen. Arch. Gynäk. **176**, 443 (1949).

HUNT, K.M.: Placental localization using the Doptone pulse recorder. J. Obstet. Gynaec. Brit. Cwlth **76**, 144 (1969).

IKLE, F.A.: Punktionsbiopsie und Beckenphlebographie zur Diagnose von Rezidiven nach Kollumkarzinom. Gynaecologia (Basel) **152**, 103 (1961).

KRATOCHWIL, A.: Der Wert der fetalen Ultraschallkardiographie in der Beurteilung der gestörten Frühschwangerschaft. Wien. klin. Wschr. **79**, 399 (1967).

KRATOCHWIL, A.: Die Ultraschall-Plazentalokalisation. Gynaecologia (Basel) **165**, 308 (1968).

KRATOCHWIL, A.: Ultraschalldiagnostik in Geburtshilfe und Gynäkologie. Stuttgart: Thieme 1968.

KRATOCHWIL, A.: Methoden und Probleme der Ultraschalldiagnostik in der Geburtshilfe und Gynäkologie. Sonderdruck aus „Elektromedizin" **14**, H. 6 (1969).

KRATOCHWIL, A.: Ein neues vaginales Ultraschall-Schnittbildverfahren. Geburtsh. u. Frauenheilk. **29**, 1573 (1969).

KRATOCHWIL, A., EISENHUT, L.: Der früheste Nachweis der fetalen Herzaktion durch Ultraschall. Geburtsh. u. Frauenheilk. **27**, 176 (1967).

KRATOCHWIL, A., HOFER, W., ALTH, G.: Zur Herdsuche in der gynäkologischen Strahlentherapie. Geburtsh. u. Frauenheilk. **31**, 833 (1971).

KRATOCHWIL, A., SCHUELLER, E.: Objektiver Nachweis von Beckenwandrezidiven nach Kollumkarzinom. Geburtsh. u. Frauenheilk. **22**, 1413 (1962).

KRATOCHWIL, A., STOEGER, H., ZEIBEKIS, N.: Darstellung von Beckenwandrezidiven im Ultraschalltomogramm. Geburtsh. u. Frauenheilk. **34**, 742 (1974).

KRATOCHWIL, A., ZEIBEKIS, N.: Die Ultraschalldiagnostik der Blasenmole. Geburtsh. u. Frauenheilk. **32**, 895 (1972).

LARSON, S.M., NELP, W.B.: Visualization of the placenta by radioisotope photoscanning using technetium 99 m-labelled albumin. Amer. J. Obstet. Gynec. **93**, 950 (1965).

LEPSIEN, POMP: Vergleichende Untersuchungen zur Ermittlung der intrauterinen Kindesgröße mit Ultraschall bei normalen und pathologischen Schwangerschaften. 69. Tagung der Nordwestdeutschen Gesellschaft für Gynäk. Bad Pyrmont, 27.–29.10.1967. Ref. in Geburtsh. u. Frauenheilk. **28**, 388 (1968).

MACHLEIDT, R., DOIL, R.: Diagnostik mit Hilfe des Ultraschalls in der Gynäkologie. Zbl. Gynäk. **42**, 1457 (1971).

MOSLER, K.H., TEICHERT, P., SCHEUER, H., MITSCHKA, F.: Ultraschallüberwachung in der Präventivgeburtshilfe. Med. Klin. **65**, 1250 (1970).

REINOLD, E.: Das Größenwachstum der Amnionhöhle in der ersten Hälfte der Gravidität. Wien. klin. Wschr. **84**, 638 (1972).

ROBERTSON, E.G., MILLAR, D.G., DAY, M.J.: Placental localization by "Colorscan" using iodine 132 labelled human serum albumin. J. Obstet. Gynaec. Brit. Cwlth **75**, 636 (1968).

RUPPIN, E., CHELIUS, H.H.: Einige Kriterien der Sonographie gynäkologischer Tumoren. Geburtsh. u. Frauenheilk. **34**, 540–550 (1974).

SCHLENSKER, K.-H.: Zur Diagnostik der vorzeitigen Lösung der normalen sitzenden Plazenta mit dem Ultraschall-Schnittbildverfahren. Geburtsh. u. Frauenheilk. **32**, 773–780 (1972).

SPECHTER, H.J.: Das „Lokalisationsgerät" und Tastzeichengerät als Hilfsmittel zur Einstellung und Dosisberechnung bei der Bewegungsbestrahlung gynäkologischer Tumoren. Strahlentherapie **103**, 571 (1957).

STEIN, W.W., HALBERSTADT, E., HEBAN, H.J.: Kasuistik intrauterin mit Ultraschall diagnostizierter Mißbildungen. 7. Dtsch. Kongr. perinatale Med., Berlin 1974.

STOEGER, H., KRATOCHWIL, A.: Ultraschallbiometrie des fetalen Wachstums. Geburtsh. u. Frauenheilk. **34**, 611–616 (1974).

SUNDEN, B.: On the diagnostic value of ultrasound in obstetrics and gynecology. Acta obstet. gynec. scand. **43**, Suppl. 6, 1 (1964).

TAYLOR, E.S., HOLMES, J.H., THOMPSON, H.E., GOTTESFELD, K.R.: Ultrasound diagnostic techniques in obstetrics and gynecology. Amer. J. Obstet. Gynec. **90**, 655 (1964).

TAYLOR, E.S., THOMPSON, H.E., GOTTESFELD, K.R., HOLMES, J.H.: Clinical use of ultrasound in obstetrics und gynecology. Amer. J. Obstet. Gynec. **99**, 671 (1967).

TAYLOR, H.C., JR.: Fetal indications for termination of pregnancy after the twenty-eight week in the presence of specific toxemia or chronic hypertension. Geburts. u. Frauenheilk. **15**, 3 (1955).

TETTI, A., TEMPORELLI, A., BALOCO, G., MASSOBRIO, M.: L'ecogramma dei tumori pelvici. Minerva ginec. **21**, 420 (1969).

THIERY, M.: Het Doppler-Effect in de Verloskunde. Ned. T. Geneesk. **24**, 354 (1968).

THOMPSON, H.: Diskussionsbemerkung. Amer. J. Obstet. Gynec. **99**, 678 (1967).

THOMPSON, H., HOLMES, J.H., GOTTESFELD, K.R., TAYLOR, E.S.: Fetal development as determined by ultrasonic pulse echo techniques. Amer. J. Obstet. Gynec. **92**, 44 (1965).

THOMPSON, H., HOLMES, J.H., GOTTESFELD, K.R., TAYLOR, E.S.: Ultrasound as a diagnostic aid in diseases of the pelvis. Amer. J. Obstet. Gynec. **98**, 472 (1967).

USHER, R., McLEAN, F.: Intrauterine growth of liveborn caucasian infants at sea level. Standards obtained from measurements in 7 dimensions of infants born between 25 and 44 weeks of gestation. Paediatrics **74**, 4 (1964).

V. MICSKY, L.T.: Ultrasonic tomography in obstetrics and gynecology. Proc. I. Int. Conf. Diagn. Ultrasound Pittsburgh 1965. New York: Plenum-Press 1966.

WEISS, P.A.M.: Typische Ultraschallbilder bei schwerer fetaler Rhesus-Erkrankung. Geburtsh. u. Frauenheilk. **34**, 640 (1974).

WEVER, H., STOCKHAUSEN, H.: Fetale Herztonkontrolle und Plazenta-Lokalisation durch Ultraschall unter Verwendung des Doppler-Effektes. Geburtsh. u. Frauenheilk. **27**, 1209 (1967).

ZACUTTI, A., BRUGNOLI, C.A.: L'impiego degli ultrasuoni nella diagnostica della tumefazioni pelviche. Minerva ginec. **22**, 772 (1970).

Subject Index

R. O. Meudt, M. Hinselmann

Ultrasonoscopic Differential Diagnosis in Obstetrics and Gynecology

Echoskopische Differential-Diagnose in Geburtshilfe und Gynäkologie
Sémiologie échoscopique en obstétrique et gynécologie
Semiologia ecoscópica en obstetricia y gynecologia
Semiologia ecoscopica in ostetricia e ginecologia
199 figs. VIII, 138 pages. 1975
ISBN 3-540-06991-7
Cloth DM 98,—
ISBN 0-387-06991-7 (North America)
Cloth $40.00

W. Wenz

Abdominal Angiography

In collaboration with G. van Kaick,
D. Beduhn, F.-J. Roth
183 figs., some in color, comprising 351 radiographs and 34 drawings
VIII, 217 pages. 1974
ISBN 3-540-06508-3
Cloth DM 72,—
ISBN 0-387-06508-3 (North America)
Cloth $27.80

Distribution rights for Japan:
Igaku Shoin Ltd., Tokyo

J. Gershon-Cohen

Atlas of Mammography

300 figs. VI, 264 pages. 1970
ISBN 3-540-05106-6
Cloth DM 120,—
ISBN 0-387-05106-6 (North America)
Cloth $33.40

A. N. Papaioannou

The Etiology of Human Breast Cancer

Endocrine Genetic, Viral, Immunologic and Other Considerations
2 figs. XII, 216 pages. 1974
ISBN 3-540-06697-7
Cloth DM 56,—
ISBN 0-387-06697-7 (North America)
Cloth $23.00

Breast Cancer: A Challenging Problem

Editors: M. L. Griem, E. V. Jensen,
J. E. Ultmann, R. W. Wissler
60 figs. 40 tab. XI, 150 pages. 1973
(Recent Results in Cancer Research, Volume 42)
ISBN 3-540-06273-4
Cloth DM 53,—
ISBN 0-387-06273-4 (North America)
Cloth $19.70

Prices are subject to change without notice

Springer-Verlag Berlin Heidelberg New York

P. Denoix

Treatment of Malignant Breast Tumors

Indications and Results
A Study Based on 1174 Cases Treated at
the Institute Gustave-Roussy between 1954
and 1962
Translator: B. Crook
18 figs. X, 92 pages. 1970 (Recent Results
in Cancer Research, Volume 31)
ISBN 3-540-04996-7
Cloth DM 58,—
ISBN 0-387-04996-7 (North America)
Cloth $19.80

P. Stoll

Gynecological Vital Cytology

Function, Microbiology, Neoplasia
Atlas of Phase-Contrast Microscopy
145 figs. VI, 81 pages. 1969
ISBN 3-540-04725-5
Cloth DM 68,—
ISBN 0-387-04725-5 (North America)
Cloth $19.80

Distribution rights for Japan:
Igaku Shoin Ltd., Tokyo

J. L. Hayward

Hormones and Human Breast Cancer

An Account of 15 Years Study
23 figs. XV, 149 pages. 1970 (Recent Results
in Cancer Research, Volume 24)
ISBN 3-540-04989-4
Cloth DM 42,—
ISBN 0-387-04989-4 (North America)
Cloth $12.10

G. Dallenbach-Hellweg

Histopathology of the Endometrium

English Translation by F. D. Dallenbach
124 figs., 2 colored plates. XI, 277 pages. 1971
ISBN 3-540-05072-8
Cloth DM 108,—
ISBN 0-387-05072-8 (North America)
Cloth $34.90

A. Labhart

Clinical Endocrinology

Theory and Practice
With a Foreword by G. W. Thorn
In collaboration with numerous experts
Translators: A. Trachsler, J. Dodsworth-
Phillips
400 figs. XXXII, 1092 pages. 1974
ISBN 3-540-06307-2
Cloth DM 125,—
ISBN 0-387-06307-2 (North America)
Cloth $48.00

Distribution rights for Japan:
Igaku Shoin Ltd., Tokyo

Diagnosis and Treatment of Fetal Disorders

Proceedings of the International Symposium
on Diagnosis and Treatment of Disorders
Affecting the Intrauterine Patient
Dorado, Puerto Rico, October 29-31, 1967
Editor: K. Adamsons
145 figs. XV, 304 pages. 1969
ISBN 3-540-04451-5
Cloth DM 76,—
ISBN 0-387-04451-5 (North America)
Cloth $14.80

Prices are subject to change without notice

Springer-Verlag
Berlin
Heidelberg
New York

Abbreviations		Abkürzungen	Abréviations	Abreviaciones	Abbreviazioni
A	aorta	Aorta	aorte	aorta	aorta
B	bladder	Blase	vessie	vejiga	vescica
B₁	initial echo (front parietal bone)	Initialecho (vorderes Os parietale)	êcho initial (os pariétal antérieur)	eco inicial (pared anterior del cranéo)	eco iniziale (osso parietale anteriore)
B₂	final echo (rear parietal bone)	Endecho (hinteres Os parietale)	écho final (os pariétal postérieur)	eco final (pared posterior del cranéo)	eco finale (osso parietale posteriore)
BD	abdominal wall	Bauchdecke	paroi abdominale	pared abdominal	parete addominale
BL	vesicular mole	Blasenmole	môle hydatiforme	mola vesicular	mola vescicolare
COV	cystic ovarian tumor	cystischer Ovarialtumor	tumeur ovarienne cystique	quiste de ovario	tumore ovarico cistico
D	intestinal echo	Darmecho	écho intestinal	ecos del intestino	eco di derivazione intestinale
FB	gestational sac	Fruchtblase	cavité amniotique	cavidad amniótica	sacco amniotico
FH	uterine cavity	Fruchthöhle	cavité amniotique	cavidad amniótica	cavo amniotico
FL	liquid blood	flüssiges Blut	sang liquide	heamatoma retro-placentario (sangre no coagulada)	sangue non ancora coagulato
FO	fronto-occipital diameter	frontooccipitaler Durchmesser	diam. fronto-occipital	diámetro fronto occipital	diametro fronto-occipitale
FW	amniotic fluid	Fruchtwasser	liquide amniotique	líquido amniótico	liquido amniotico
HW	posterior wall	Hinterwand	paroi postérieure	pared posterior	parete posteriore
K	head	Kopf	tête	cabeza	testa
KL	small parts	kleine Teile	partie foetales	extremidades des fetales	estremità fetali
LI	left kidney	linke Niere	rein gauche	riñón izquierdo	rene sinistro
M	myoma	Myom	myome	mioma	mioma
M₁	subserosal myomic nodules	subseröse Myomknoten	noeuds myomateux sous-séreux	mioma subseroso	noduli miomatosi sottosierosi
M₂	cervical myoma	Cervixmyom	myome du col de l'uterus	mioma cervical	mioma cervicale
ME	central echo	Mittelecho	écho médian	eco medio	eco mediano
N	necrotic material	Nekrosematerial	matières de nécrose	zona de necrosis	materiale necrotico
O	base point	Basispunkt	point de base	punto inicial	punto di base
P	portio	Portio	portion	cuello uterino	portio uterina
PL	placenta	Placenta	placenta	placenta	placenta
PM	partially denatur-ated chorionic villi and severely macerated fetus	entartete Chorion-zotten und stark macerierter Fetus	villosités placen-taires dégénérees et foetus fortement macéré	feto macerado y vesiculas de vellosidades coriónicas	villi coriali par-zialmente degene-rati e feto grave-mente macerato
PR	promontorium	Promontorium	promontoire	promontorio	promontorio
RE	right kidney	rechte Niere	rein droit	riñón derecho	rene destro
RU	torso	Rumpf	tronc	cuerpo	tronco
S	symphysis	Symphyse	symphyse	sinfisis	sinfisi
SP	Spaldings sign and double contouring of cranium	Spalding und Doppelkontur des Schädels	Spalding et double contoure du crâne	signo de Spalding	segno di Spalding e doppio contorno del cranio
U	uterus	Uterus	utérus	útero	utero
WS	spinal column	Wirbelsäule	colonne vertébrale	columna vertebral	colonna vertebrale
X	xiphoid	Xiphoid	xiphoide	xiphoïde	xifoide

Abbreviations   Abkürzungen   Abréviations   Abreviaciones   Abbreviazioni